The COVID-19 Pandemic and Long-Term Care

This important book examines how nursing homes experienced the COVID-19 pandemic, how it affected the residents and staff, and how the industry can be reformed to better meet the demands of a similar health crisis in the future.

Data-led and richly illustrated with insightful charts throughout, the book begins with a thorough overview of what occurred in nursing homes during the pandemic, situated within a broader perspective of the regulatory system in which long-term care operates in different regions of the world. It then moves on to detail those issues that made managing nursing homes during the pandemic so challenging, before providing an insightful analysis into how nursing homes can reform their policies and practices ahead of a possible future pandemic.

Written by a gerontological nurse and Director of Nursing with over 30 years of experience in the long-term care industry, this book will interest researchers and practitioners across public health and nursing.

Delia Marie Franklin is a registered nurse who has over 40 years of experience in the healthcare profession, including approximately eight years of experience as a Director of Nursing in the long-term care industry. As a nurse, her knowledge base of long-term care and gerontological nursing is intertwined with educational materials establishing a broader understanding of the COVID-19 pandemic, its impact on nursing homes worldwide, and the multifactorial systems needed for culture change and reform in the industry.

The COVID-19 Pandemic and Long-Term Care
Insights for Reform

Delia Marie Franklin

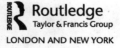
Routledge
Taylor & Francis Group

LONDON AND NEW YORK

First published 2025
by Routledge
4 Park Square, Milton Park, Abingdon, Oxon OX14 4RN

and by Routledge
605 Third Avenue, New York, NY 10158

Routledge is an imprint of the Taylor & Francis Group, an informa business

British Library Cataloguing-in-Publication Data
A catalogue record for this book is available from the British Library

ISBN: 978-1-032-73833-8 (hbk)
ISBN: 978-1-032-73839-0 (pbk)
ISBN: 978-1-003-46619-2 (ebk)

DOI: 10.4324/9781003466192

Typeset in Times New Roman
by Apex CoVantage, LLC

The COVID-19 Pandemic and Long-Term Care: Insights for Reform is dedicated to all of the residents and LTC employees who lost their lives during the pandemic.

Contents

Figures

Introduction—The COVID-19 Pandemic and Long-Term Care: Insights for Reform

Many of the educational materials presented in this book are based on the employment experiences of nurses during the COVID-19 pandemic. Nurses working as a Director of Nursing in a skilled nursing facility, when the COVID-19 pandemic initiated in the United States, elicited a career experience that will be remembered for decades by nurses throughout the globe.

In one California facility, a conversation between the facility dietician and nurses about the Diamond Princess cruise ship that was quarantined due to SARS-CoV-2 occurred a couple of weeks prior to the Centers for Disease Control and Prevention (CDC) and Centers for Medicare & Medicaid Services (CMS) instituting mitigation protocols in nursing homes and elicited concern among employees. We now know that the cruise ship stayed in Yokohama, Japan, and during the month of quarantine, approximately 700 individuals were infected and nine people died. In addition, by June 2020, over 40 cruise ships had experienced confirmed COVID-19-positive cases.

In early January 2020, healthcare workers (HCWs) had no knowledge base of what the medical community would be experiencing for years related to a pandemic. Even nurses who had over 40 years of experience soon realized that no amount of education or experience really prepared them for the oncoming challenges that nursing homes would face. By February 23, 2020, there were 14 confirmed COVID-19 cases in the United States and 39 additional positive cases that entailed citizens returning from China and the Diamond Princess cruise ship.

The World Health Organization (WHO) declared the COVID-19 outbreak to be a pandemic in March 2020. On March 13, 2020, CMS, on the basis of CDC recommendations, issued a memorandum restricting visitors, nonessential personnel and communal activities, and instituting COVID screening processes in American nursing homes. This essentially was the beginning of multiple received memorandums, policies, protocols, procedures, practices, surveillances, testing, and data collection processes that would be implemented in nursing homes nationally.

By February 2022, a Kaiser Family Foundation article reported that there were over 200,000 deaths of residents and staff in skilled nursing facilities

DOI: 10.4324/9781003466192-1

since the initiation of the pandemic; this number encompassed 23% of all COVID-19 deaths in the United States. By December 2023, there were over a million deaths in the United States and almost seven million deaths globally from SARS-CoV-2. The loss of human life is the most devastating consequence of the virus and will impact populations in communities, countries, and the long-term care (LTC) industry for years to come.

Because of so many adversities experienced in nursing homes within countries due to COVID, this book was formulated to assist in mitigation for future pandemics. The COVID-19 pandemic and its impact on the nursing home industry, HCWs, patients, families, and communities are explored to assist in gaining broader insights about viral pandemics. Through careful assessment and discussion, new information can be explored to assist the LTC industry, governments, and organizations with system, policy, structural, and governmental changes needed for improved quality of elder care services globally.

For one, a lot of nursing homes are not structurally built to provide for effective red COVID units in their facilities. Having a safe entrance and exit area on a COVID unit that can be isolated from the remainder of the facility poses a challenge in some facilities. Staffing is a second challenge in these institutions; the healthcare profession and its many different branches worldwide have a staffing challenge without a pandemic, add the multifaceted dynamics that develop with pandemic protocols and numerous other adversities can evolve. In addition, mandated education on pandemics needs to be implemented to assist HCWs in better understanding of infection prevention and control (IPC) policies, their role in providing care for patients during a public health emergency (PHE), and protocols for the deterrence of spreading pathogens in the employment environment.

Other avenues discussed to enhance elder care provisions include the structural, policy, and procedural changes for improvement of surveillance, mitigation, and quality of care; regulatory systems and changes in protocols to prepare for future pandemics; governmental strategies for advancement of healthcare delivery in LTC; LTC facility structural and internal changes for elder care provisions; deinstitutionalization of nursing homes; and the organizations globally that assist in pandemic preparation plans. Through exploring these many different reform strategies, we can build on mitigation improvement with regard to the next PHE.

Section I

COVID-19 in Nursing Homes and Its Impacts

1 Nursing Home Susceptibility for Transmission

Residents and Employees

When the WHO declared the COVID-19 pandemic, it initiated a chain of events that had not been implemented in the United States since the Spanish Flu of 1918. Social distancing, mask mandates, and isolative precautions with a complete nationwide and worldwide lockdown occurred almost overnight. It impacted every country, every culture, every state, every city, every community, and every person globally.

March 2020 also instituted a new ongoing medical dilemma for nursing homes that had not been encountered previously, at least not during the careers of the current population of HCWs. As gerontological nurses, we had never seen or experienced a total systematic restructuring of the medical profession, nursing homes, hospitals, and medical offices during our years employed in the profession. The pandemic evolved into a fast-paced learning curve on worldwide infection processes that occurred in a very short time frame, impacting all branches of medicine.

As an industry, LTC proved to be ground zero for COVID-19. In nursing homes, there have been multiple internal and external factors identified for the ongoing transmission of SARS-CoV-2, and some of these pre-COVID elements in the industry disproportionately greatly affected gerontological clients.

Internal and External Factors Affecting Transmission Rates

Internal factors are elements that can be eradicated or minimized by establishing management strategies to decrease transmission risk potential. Some internal factors in nursing homes are staffing numbers; cohabitation; admissions; personnel being employed at multiple facilities; resident-shared toileting, water, and dining; and asymptomatic transmissions.

However, external factors that may impact transmission rates in LTC occur outside of the facility and generally cannot be controlled or managed by

DOI: 10.4324/9781003466192-3

employees. External factors can encompass urban location, community transmission rates, facility size, and personal protective equipment (PPE) availability. Several news articles have been published globally about how COVID exposed an already broken nursing home industry. There are many factors identified in the articles that were potentially linked to the SARS-CoV-2 crisis in LTC; one of those dynamics is staffing.

Employees

Before the pandemic, staffing was an ongoing problem in elder care environments. The increased workload and healthcare provider positive COVID-19 cases exacerbated that shortage. All departments in nursing homes fell short at times, because of the pandemic, and staffing shortages still existed in 2024. It is well acknowledged that employee shortages can potentially contribute to viral transmission related to improper infection control practices, due to time constraints.

It has also been identified that low employee wages in elder care environments limit staff availability and at times contribute to decreased resident quality of care. Some organizations have suggested that a restructuring of employee wages in the LTC industry could potentially improve the provision of healthcare services for gerontological clients; this will be elaborated on in more detail later.

Worldwide, SARS-CoV-2 continues to enter nursing homes; outbreaks continue today through various transmission sources. Some studies revealed that a larger employee pool size and healthcare providers working in multiple facilities contribute to higher coronavirus transmission rates. Additionally, it has been identified that asymptomatic employees were the root cause of most initial nursing home transmissions and outbreaks, and that populace and facility structure are additional contributing factors.

Populace and Facility Structure

Facility size, urban location, and community COVID rates are all intertwined; the larger the populace, the increased chance for initial and ongoing viral transmissions. According to Statista by October 5, 2022, the states with the highest number of COVID-19 cases were California, Texas, Florida, and New York.[1] And, Worldometer in July 2022 identified the United States, India, Brazil, France, and Germany as the countries with the highest number of positive coronavirus cases.[2] Figure 1.1 depicts the number of nursing homes impacted by COVID-19 in specific American states.

A few studies stated that the correlation between COVID-19 transmission and a facility's 5-star rating or previous nursing home infection control deficiencies were not predictive factors of SARS-CoV-2 entering a facility. Other

March 2021: Number of US Nursing Homes Impacted by COVID

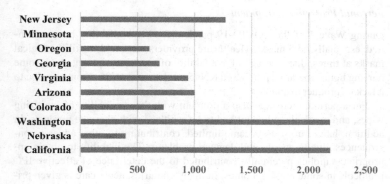

Figure 1.1 Number of US Nursing Homes COVID Impacted by March 2021.[3]

Source: The COVID Tracking Project. This is a bar graph that contains a horizontal axis listing numbers from 0 to 2,500 and a vertical axis listing specific US states depicting the number of nursing homes impacted by COVID in 2021; there were below 500 facilities in Nebraska and above 2,000 in Washington.

studies, such as the one in 2020, that sampled 8,943 nursing homes in 23 American states and the District of Columbia revealed that rates of deficiencies and complaints defined as failures to meet compliance standards or allegations of noncompliance with federal requirements were higher in nursing homes that reported cases of coronavirus.[4]

Cohabitation and the sharing of restrooms, shower rooms, and dining were all also relayed as possible contributing factors to ongoing SARS-CoV-2 transmission in care homes. Most post-acute facilities are structured with dual or multiple occupancy rooms, with a limited number of private rooms for skilled admissions. Potential reforms to address the architectural designs of nursing homes will be discussed in Chapter 5. Additionally, residents with a cognitive impairment are more prone to infections.

Residents

In one IMPACT medical review, 5,200 records of nursing homes in 25 states were assessed for residents who expired within 30 days of a COVID diagnosis. The analysis revealed that individuals with moderate or severe cognitive impairment were twice as likely to die from COVID, as those with mild or no cognitive impairment.[5] Dementia was identified as a predictor of susceptibility to an infection related to mask noncompliance and other infection control practices, such as hand hygiene. Additionally, there were problems with obtaining PPE at the initiation of the pandemic in many nursing homes.

Personal Protective Equipment

During Wave 1 of the COVID-19 pandemic, PPE availability became limited, especially N95 masks. Healthcare providers were told to utilize surgical masks at times, due to a lack of availability of proper equipment. And, some nursing home operators purchased KN95 masks versus N95 respirators due to a lack of product availability.

For a period, there was also a problem with the availability of sanitizing wipes, and medical equipment had to be sanitized with alternate products. In addition, hand sanitizers became limited, contributing to other adverse consequences, due to supply and demand problems. The inability to obtain appropriate supplies potentially contributed to the deterrence of effective IPC protocols in some nursing homes. In many countries, acute care is given priority over LTC, thus limiting the PPE supply in nursing homes even more adversely, potentially contributing to increased outbreaks.

Morbidity and Mortality

As of July 2024, the Centers for Medicare & Medicaid Services (CMS) in the United States reported that there had been 2,047,225 positive resident COVID cases identified and 171,588 resident deaths in nursing home facilities nationwide.[6] Gerontological clients have a higher risk factor for mortality in pandemic situations, due to compromised immune systems (as we age the immune system is slower to respond) and comorbidity. The SARS-CoV-2 virus has proven to be more virulent with obesity, diabetes, heart disease, chronic kidney disease, and lung disease. One study identified that there was a 92.8% risk of mortality with at least one comorbidity.[7] Figure 1.2 illustrates state-specific positive COVID cases in nursing homes in the United States.

In a White House Briefing in February of 2022, President Biden stated,

> The pandemic has highlighted the tragic impact of substandard conditions at nursing homes, which are home to many of our most at-risk community members. More than 1.4 million people live in over 15,500 Medicare and Medicaid certified nursing homes across the nation. In the past two years, more than 200,000 residents and staff have died from COVID-19, nearly a quarter of all coronavirus deaths in the United States.[8]

As of July 2024, it was identified that 1,875,635 residents have recovered from coronavirus in US nursing homes, based on CMS statistics. In addition, many of the 1,918,630 US employees in LTC facilities that tested positive for COVID have also recovered.[10]

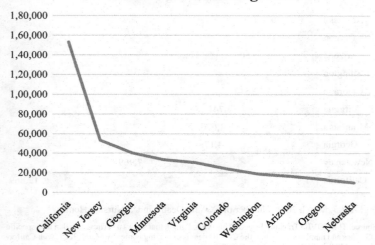

March 2021: Number of Positive COVID Cases in US Nursing Homes

Figure 1.2 Number of Positive COVID Cases in US Nursing Homes, 2021.[9]

Source: The COVID Tracking Project. This is a line graph that illustrates a vertical axis of numbers from 0 to 180,000 and a horizontal axis listing specific US states that shows the 2021 number of positive COVID cases in nursing homes, revealing California with the highest number of cases at 153,172 and Nebraska at the lowest with 9,975 cases.

An American Association of Retired Persons (AARP) report on Nebraska nursing homes revealed that 95% of all their facilities had confirmed positive cases of COVID-19 since the beginning of the pandemic. And, for the last 30-day reporting period in 2021, nursing home deaths comprised 54% of all COVID deaths in Nebraska, further stating, "As COVID-19 brings to light long-standing flaws in the nation's long-term care system. AARP's Public Policy Institute has unveiled a new report, *COVID-19 and Nursing Home Residents* that contains a series of strategies to improve the quality of long-term services and supports."[11] In Figure 1.3, the specific state deaths in LTC homes are identified.

Other Countries

The European Centre for Disease Prevention and Control (ECDC) established surveillance of COVID-19 outbreaks (TESSy) in nursing/care homes within the European Union (EU) and European Economic Area (EEA) countries including Austria, Belgium, Croatia, Cyprus, Denmark, France, Germany,

March 2021: Number of COVID Deaths in US Nursing Homes

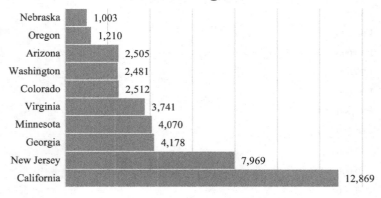

Figure 1.3 March 2021: Number of COVID Deaths in US Nursing Homes.[12]

Source: The COVID Tracking Project. This is a bar graph that shows a vertical axis that lists specific US states and numbers, revealing the COVID deaths in nursing homes by March 2021, with California at 12,869 and Nebraska totaling 1,003 deaths.

Ireland, Italy, Lithuania, Luxembourg, Netherlands, Norway, Portugal, Slovenia, Spain, and Sweden in January 2021.

There are approximately 2.9 million residents in 43,000 facilities within EU and EEA countries.[13] By June 30, 2020, more than 80,000 deaths related to COVID-19 had occurred in European elder care homes.[14] The WHO issued a policy brief in July 2020, that revealed in many countries evidence showed that more than 40% of SARS-CoV-2-related deaths had been linked to LTC facilities, with figures being as high as 80% in some high-income countries.[15] In Figure 1.4, the number of positive coronavirus cases in nursing homes within the EU is illustrated from January to November 2021.

Neil Gandal, a Tel Aviv University researcher, reported that he assessed 32 European countries and found a correlation between the number of nursing/elder care home beds and mortality rates from COVID. The countries in his study with the highest SARS-CoV-2 death rates were the United Kingdom, Italy, Spain, and Belgium. He stated, "I see a clear pattern, with fewer deaths in countries where elderly people tend to live with families, and high mortality rates in countries that heavily rely on care homes."[17]

Belgium's nursing homes have accounted for 57% of all COVID mortality (11,369 residents as of January 2022) in this country.[18] The Italian Institute for Health (ISS) provided the first available dataset on SARS-CoV-2 cases in Italy from February to May 2020; it was estimated that the overall mortality

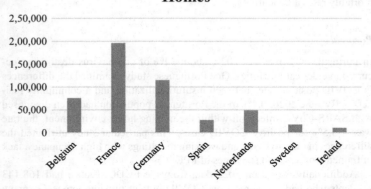

Figure 1.4 Number of Positive COVID Cases in EU Nursing Homes, 2021.[16]

Source: European Centre for Disease Prevention and Control. This is a column graph that depicts a vertical axis of numbers from 0 to 250,000 and a horizontal axis that lists specific countries, revealing positive COVID cases in EU nursing homes in 2021, with France having over 150,000 cases and Ireland having under 50,000.

rate was 9.1% in Italian nursing homes and that 41% of the deaths during this period were COVID-related.[19] By January 2021, 14,066 SARS-CoV-2 diagnosed deaths in nursing homes had occurred, accounting for 27% of Germany's mortality rate.[20]

Many other countries had similar statistics regarding their nursing home population. In Canada, it was estimated in 2021 that 69% of their COVID deaths were linked to nursing homes.[21] According to the Care Quality Commission (CQC), the resident mortality toll from COVID-19 in England's elder care homes was 19,248 in 2020, 11,472 in 2021, 4,332 in July 2022, and 1,141 as of September 2023.[22]

France

A French investigation of the correlation between the external pressure (community rates) of COVID-19 and outbreaks in the nursing homes in the Auvergne-Rhone-Alpes region revealed a definitive association between the two. It was identified that 52% of the facilities in the region had outbreaks that lasted 11–21 days after positive cases were identified in the surrounding populace.[23] Some elder care facilities in France instituted voluntary confinement of staff in the facilities with their residents, and analysis of this mitigation process demonstrated that this intervention did indeed subdue the transmission of the virus. It is estimated that 44% of coronavirus deaths in France occurred in LTC facilities.[24] In Figure 1.5, January to November 2021 global LTC resident mortality rates are identified.

Portugal

In Portugal, by November 2020, about 34% of coronavirus deaths had occurred in elder care facilities. One Portuguese study examined the differences in COVID positive rates between institutionalization and a community residence. By June 2020, 0.4% of the Portuguese population had been diagnosed with SARS-CoV-2 infection; within the nursing home environment, the rate was at 3.5% for positive COVID cases. This particular study attributed the differences in rates to living and working in settings with high occupancy, lack of trained workers, and shortages of PPE.[26]

Additionally, based on 2022 data from the ECDC, France had 168,143 residents who had recovered from COVID in their nursing homes, Germany had 89,852 residents who had recovered, the Netherlands had 39,774 residents who had recovered from COVID-19, and Sweden had 11,782 positive SARS-CoV-2 residents who had survived in elder care facilities.[27] Not only were there the adversities of mortality and morbidity, but there were also other psychological and physical burdens for LTC residents.

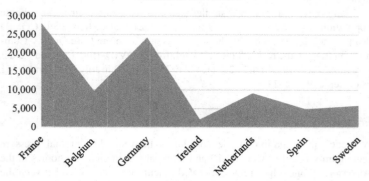

Global Mortality Numbers in Nursing Homes in 2021

Figure 1.5 Global Resident Mortality Numbers in 2021.[25]

Source: European Centre for Disease Prevention and Control. This is an area graph that contains a vertical axis of numbers from 0 to 30,000 and a horizontal axis listing specific countries, portraying the number of global mortalities by 2021, with France having over 25,000 deaths and Sweden having under 5,000 deaths.

Additional Burdens Experienced by Customers

During the initial US lockdown of nursing homes in March 2020, many family members and patients were distraught over the inability to be able to visit with each other in-person. And, when SARS-CoV-2 actually transmitted into nursing homes, the problems were multiplied due to illness, potential and/or actual death of patients, and the inability to provide in-person familial emotional and psychological support.

Articles published on the effects of the pandemic on the mental health of residents discussed both gerontological clients with no pre-existing mental health issue identified and those residents with pre-pandemic psychiatric diagnosis established, and how the pandemic restrictions either generated new symptoms or exacerbated preceding psychological symptomatology.

Discussing the pandemic's psychological and physical burdens experienced by customers in the LTC industry, including depression, anxiety, social isolation, post-traumatic stress disorder (PTSD), decline in functional ability, weight loss, falls, exacerbation of behaviors (anger/aggression), and pressure injuries (PIs) can assist in understanding additional consequences of pandemics in nursing homes.

Psychological Burdens

Initially, in US nursing homes at the beginning of the pandemic, almost complete social isolation related to in-person contact was implemented; all residents were restricted to their rooms. Staff were pretty much the only source of in-person contact for residents and that situation lasted for a long period of time. Eventually, window visits with family members were initiated, but prior to CMS granting permission for this process to occur, electronic contact/communication (texting, phone calls, facetime, zoom, etc.) was the only source for familial correspondence utilized by most patients. And, even when hall bingo or hall karaoke was initiated, there was still the social distancing that needed to be maintained at 6 feet for all residents, limiting human contact in facilities.

Loneliness and Failure to Thrive

It is well established that social isolation can lead to mental and physical health decline. A study published in the *Journal of American Medical Directors Association* on the association between social connection (social support, social engagement, social network, and loneliness) and mental health outcomes identified that with limited social connection, there was an increased probability of depression; responsive behaviors; mood, affect, and emotions being impacted; anxiety; increased medication use; cognitive decline; boredom; suicidal ideation; psychiatric morbidity; and daily crying.[28] It is further established that social isolation and loneliness can also have a negative impact on the physical health status of nursing home residents including cardiovascular disease and high blood pressure and can lead to increased mortality. A survey conducted in the United States from July to August 2020, which received responses from 365 LTC residents, revealed that loneliness and failure to thrive exacerbated during the pandemic, decreasing resident quality of life. The following are statistical percentages from that survey:

1. Only 5% of respondents reported having visitors three or more times per week, compared with 56% before the outbreak.
2. Only 28% reported that they went outside to enjoy fresh air one or more times per week, compared with 83% before the outbreak.
3. 54% reported that they were not participating in any in-home organized activities, compared with 14% before the outbreak.
4. Only 13% reported eating their meals in the dining room, compared with 69% before the outbreak.[29]

Additionally, 76% of the respondents reported that they felt lonelier under the restrictions, an unsurprising finding given that 64% of residents indicated that they no longer even left their rooms to socialize with other residents.[30]

An analysis in Ireland, which examined the psychosocial impact of COVID-19 nursing home restrictions on visitors, identified that family members that assisted in providing caregiving to their loved ones prior to the pandemic reported significantly lower psychological and emotional well-being:

• 38% stated the restrictions had a significant negative impact on communication with staff.
• 27% reported decreased satisfaction with care provided.
• 49% stated that their loved one was not coping well with the restrictions.[31]

Social connection is an important aspect in deterring psychological burdens in LTC, not only for the resident but also for caregivers and/or family members. Due to the identified mental health consequences experienced by residents and family members that included anxiety and depression, we need to evaluate the protocols for future pandemics and formulate solutions that promote mental well-being in the LTC industry.

Depression and Anxiety

In a 2020 report from the Kaiser Family Foundation, it was revealed that, in Washington, almost half of the residents had experienced depression or depressive symptoms.[32] Another study, which encompassed an evaluation of the Minimum Data Set (a resident assessment form that is submitted for Medicare and Medicaid reimbursement) in Connecticut nursing homes for 2021, revealed the following:

We found that nursing home resident outcomes worsened on a broad array of measures. The prevalence of depressive symptoms increased by six percentage points relative to before the pandemic in the beginning of March-representing a 15% increase. The share of residents with unplanned substantial weight loss also increased by six percentage points relative to the beginning of March-representing a 150% increase. We also found significant increases in episodes of incontinence (four percentage points) and significant reductions in cognitive functioning. Our findings suggest that loneliness and isolation play an important role.[33]

Grief associated with the COVID-19 pandemic is another factor that can manifest depressive symptoms. Residents could experience sadness and other symptoms of depression at any point in the grieving process. On the basis of empirical findings, Melanie Vachon and her colleagues developed a definition of *"pandemic grief"*—neither normal nor "complicated," pandemic grief is a hushed mourning process suspended in time, punctuated by public health measures, with little social recognition for the suffering it causes.[34]

It has been identified that the COVID-19 pandemic was a "tsunami of loss" for residents and staff, and that, during the pandemic, grief had taken on different meanings for residents due to the sheer number of people dying in close congregate settings and the inability to say proper goodbyes or hold funeral services, due to isolative practices. Also, some psychologists and psychiatrists relayed that residents had reported increased anxiety related to fear of contracting COVID, witnessing other residents and staff contract COVID, and some contracting COVID themselves.

Other countries exhibited some similar results; even before the COVID-19 pandemic, almost half of the residents in German nursing homes showed signs of depressive symptoms. And, the coronavirus restrictions were accompanied by increased negative consequences regarding the health of German LTC residents.[35]

Anxiety is explained as intense, excessive, and persistent worry and fear about everyday situations. In France and the Netherlands, where similar COVID restrictions applied, increased anxiety, depression, loneliness, and an increase in behavioral problems were observed.[36] Residents without cognitive impairment seemed to be the most affected, as illustrated in Figure 1.6. During the COVID-19 measures in the Netherlands, it was identified that the well-being of gerontological LTC residents was severely affected; six to ten weeks after the implementation of the visitor ban, high levels of loneliness, depression, and a significant exacerbation in mood and behavioral problems were reported.[37]

A study in Thailand revealed that most residents reported a moderate or severe impact from COVID-19 related to economic reasons. In the study, 70% of residents reported no or mild psychological stress from COVID-19; however, 5.5% had post-traumatic stress, 7.0% had depression, and 12.0% had

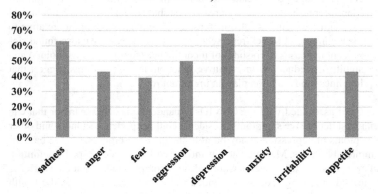

Figure 1.6 Percentage of LTC Resident Increased Mental Health Symptomatology.[39]

Source: *J Am Med Dir Assoc.* This is a column graph illustrating vertical axis percentages from 0% to 80% and a horizontal axis listing resident mood and behavioral changes related to COVID, with sadness and depression being the highest percentages.

anxiety. Higher psychological stress from COVID-19 and having respiratory tract infection symptoms were independently associated with post-traumatic stress, depression, and anxiety. And, receiving COVID-19 news via social media was independently associated with post-traumatic stress and depression symptoms.[38]

Post-Traumatic Stress Disorder

PTSD is a mental health condition that is triggered by a traumatic event wherein the symptoms get worse, last for months or years, and interfere with day-to-day functioning. Given the enormous impact of COVID-19 on the vulnerable gerontological population, it is crucial to explore its effects on all aspects of their mental health, including post-traumatic stress-like symptoms.

An assessment in Spain reported that 6.81% of people from the elderly age group were suffering from PTSD during the COVID-19 pandemic.[40] Another study in France revealed a 9.9% incidence of PTSD in the elderly age group surviving the coronavirus illness.[41]

In an analysis in China, 26.9% of gerontological adults surviving COVID-19 had PTSD symptoms, with intrusion symptoms in 30.8% of the cases, avoidance symptoms in 30.8%, and hyperarousal symptoms in 30.8% of the sampled individuals.[42] In addition, a study conducted in Ireland concluded that 1.6% of the elderly population subjects had COVID-19-related PTSD.[43] This article revealed that most of the studies link an association between being of the female gender to a higher incidence of PTSD.

An existing psychiatric illness was also a significant risk factor for the development of COVID-19-associated PTSD. One study found that out of 33.5% of patients with a pre-existing psychiatric condition, 6.5% had developed PTSD by the four-week follow-up medical visit.[44] There was also exacerbation of residents' mood and behavior in nursing homes worldwide during the pandemic.

Exacerbation of Behaviors: Anger and Aggression

A Virginia nursing home clinician survey revealed that 74% of participants saw behavioral symptoms related to dementia sharply increase during the pandemic, including irritability, aggression, disinhibition, delusions, hallucinations, and mania.[45]

A 2023 analysis conducted on neuropsychiatric symptoms revealed that France found an increase in hallucinations during the lockdown in residents diagnosed with Alzheimer's disease.[46] A German nursing homes study identified a 16.9% increase in aggression and a 16.9% increase in wandering with dementia residents during the pandemic.[47] In yet another study, neuropsychiatric symptoms of apathy, anxiety, anger, and agitation were the most identified and increased in occurrence, being associated with adverse cognitions, mainly triggered by protracted isolation.[48]

LTC facilities (199 professionals) in the Netherlands participated in an evaluation of resident behaviors and reported opposite results, 77% of participants observed a decrease in challenging behavior among residents with advanced dementia, due to the decrease in stimuli.

However, there was an increase in challenging behavior among most residents without dementia, observed by 66% of the individuals who participated in the survey, and 43% of professionals felt that residents with mild dementia had an increase in adverse behaviors (psychotic, agitated, or apathetic).[49] And, a Maltese LTC facility reported that restrictions increased challenging behaviors with residents, especially agitation and aggression.[50]

Physical Burdens

Weight Loss

Significant unplanned weight loss was another adversity during the pandemic lockdown, not only for residents who were diagnosed with COVID-19 but also for individuals who never contracted the virus. There are multifactorial dynamics identified for the increased weight loss in LTC facilities; for those residents who tested positive for COVID-19, the loss of weight can be attributed to fever; inflammation; loss of appetite and taste; fatigue; functional decline; general malnutrition; and endocrine, cardiac, and renal dysfunction. Also, the isolation decreased activity levels, and potential staggering of meal times may well have contributed to increased weight loss for other residents in nursing homes.

An analysis from March 1, 2020, to May 31, 2020, in a 200-bed nursing home located in Chicago, Illinois, revealed a 4.6% weight loss in positive COVID residents and a 2.4% weight loss in residents without SARS-CoV-2.[51] Another study that evaluated resident weights in an urban LTC facility from December 2019 to April 2020 revealed that 67% of the residents lost weight and 23% lost over 5% of their body weight.[52] In addition, residents residing in nursing homes in Connecticut experienced adverse consequences during the pandemic with unplanned significant weight loss doubling in comparison to previous years.[53]

An analysis of 317 residents (111 residents were COVID-positive and survived) in nursing homes in France during Wave 1 of the pandemic revealed a weight loss above 5% in 32% of the individuals within a three-month time period.[54] Four European LTC facilities were evaluated for the impact of COVID-19 on residents during Wave I, with weight loss observed in 38.4% of the residents, and the nutritional assessment conducted by dietary worsened in 92.9% of residents whose previous nutritional situation was considered normal,[55] further stating:

> The findings of this study show that institutionalized older adults presented significant worsening in their functional, cognitive, emotional, and nutritional status after the first wave of the pandemic, regardless of whether they were infected by SARS-CoV-2 or not, since no clinically or statistically significant differences were found between the two groups.[56]

Falls

Injuries from falls were an ongoing concern in many facilities prior to COVID; approximately one-third of gerontological people living in nursing homes fall at least once per year, with half of them experiencing multiple falls.[57] The implemented isolation precautions that generated the eradication of group dining, group activities, and general reduction of resident physical activity added additional challenges for LTC staff. Potential deconditioning, muscle wasting, increased weakness, and balance problems can contribute to increased falls.

Falls did increase in many elder care facilities during the pandemic, partly due to resident cognitive and physical decline. A study conducted involving three Nebraska nursing homes demonstrated a 72% increase in resident falls from 2019 to 2020.[58] An assessment (between February and May 2020) of adverse events in Italian nursing homes that included falls revealed 1,841 incidents that occurred regarding residents in 444 LTC facilities.[59] Falls in nursing homes in Ontario, Canada, have been increasing over the years (their benchmark score is 9%); in 2011, the average score for their facilities was 14.1%, and in 2021, it was 16.7%.[60]

Pressure Injuries

The development of PIs in LTC facilities has been a reoccurring sentinel event identified by CMS for years. PIs range in severity from stage I (non-blanchable redness) to stage IV (exposed muscle, tendons, ligaments, and/or bone tissue) and develop due to a wide range of factors. In nursing homes, comorbidities, systemic and nutritional decline, incontinence, and the aging process that results in the thinning of skin are all risk factors for the development of PIs.

A Nebraska study of three nursing homes during the pandemic demonstrated no increase in the development of PIs in the 2019 (22 PIs) to 2020 (21 PIs) comparison.[61] Quarterly CMS data in the United States indicate that PIs in LTC facilities increased by 31% between the 2018 fourth quarter and the 2021 second quarter in the United States.[62] And, a 2023 study across Organization for Economic Co-Operation and Development (OECD) countries noted that the observed median prevalence of pressure ulcers in LTC units was 5.4%. The highest prevalence rates were observed in Spain (9.7%), Italy (9.9%), and Portugal (13.1%).[63]

Furthermore, a LTC facility in Chicago, Illinois, was fined $25,000 in the first quarter of 2022 for failing to perform a comprehensive skin assessment and to prevent the development of a PI.[64] In addition, a nursing home in Berwyn, Illinois, was fined $25,000 for failing to ensure that residents were free from neglect by failing to prevent PIs.[65]

Additionally, COVID-19 took a tremendous toll on the medical community and HCWs, generating psychological and physical burdens for employees in the industry.

Impact on HCWs

On top of staffing shortages and burn-out, there were other physical and psychological burdens for HCWs including depression, anxiety, and PTSD. And, HCWs were not the only employees who faced adverse consequences during the pandemic, housekeeping, dietary, social services, activities, administration, maintenance, rehabilitation, and medical records were also impacted.

Staffing Shortages

We elaborated briefly on this issue earlier, but we will examine the topic more in-depth at this time. The COVID enforced regulations and protocols that facilitated the loss of external agencies and family caregivers, added additional impacts that were detrimental to both staff and residents. Staffing shortages contribute to burnout, and burnout contributes to staff turnover, which perpetuates more stress. It is a vicious cycle that was multiplied by the pandemic.

Statistics

A *Nursing in the time of COVID-19* report found that 34% of nurses reported that it was very likely they would leave their job by the end of 2022; 44% stated that burnout and high-stress environments were the main factors behind their decisions, and 32% of nurses who planned to quit their positions intended to leave the nursing field or retire.[66] Another study of nursing homes in the United States revealed that there were reported shortages of licensed nurses, nurse aides, clinical staff, and other staff. Georgia and Minnesota had the highest rates of shortages with regard to licensed nurses and nurse aides, both at 25%.[67]

Increased nurse shortages were also noted around the globe during the COVID-19 pandemic.

In the United Kingdom, the National Health Service (NHS) carried nearly 40,000 nurse vacancies, and 36% of the current workforce considered leaving in 2021.[68] In the early stages of the pandemic in South Korea, more than 10% of its nurses reported intentions to quit.[69] Research findings in both the Philippines and Pakistan showed that burnout and prolonged stress were predictors of turnover intentions among nurses.[70] In Egypt, a 2020 study revealed that over 95% of nurses had intentions to leave their present job.[71] And, a Swedish Nurses Association survey results showed that 7% of the nursing workforce considered resigning, due to the increased pressures and workloads during the pandemic.[72]

Due to nursing shortages, aging of the nursing workforce, and growing COVID-19 effects, the International Council of Nurses estimates that up to 13 million nurses will be needed to fill the global nurse shortage gap in the future.[73] It is also estimated that by 2030, globally the medical profession will be short by 18 million HCWs.[74] And, that approximately 83 countries fail to meet the most basic standard of HCW provisions.[75]

Burnout and depression can have similar physical symptoms, but they are not the same. Burnout can lead to or exacerbate depressive episodes, but depression does not cause burnout. Depression can be related to internal factors such as chemical imbalances and may have multiple or no one definitive root cause. Burnout has a single definitive root cause, which is the physical employment environment that impacts an individual's physical and mental health.

Burnout

Burnout is characterized as a state of mental, physical, and emotional exhaustion that is related to excessive and prolonged job-related stress. Burnout is a gradual process that affects our physical and mental health in several aspects, including lowered immunity and frequent illnesses; muscle pain and frequent headaches; change in appetite and sleep patterns; isolation; fatigue; high blood pressure; gastrointestinal problems; and using food, drugs, or alcohol to cope. Anyone who feels overworked and undervalued in the employment environment is at risk for burnout. The many work-related challenges in the healthcare industry that evolved with SARS-CoV-2 contributed to increased caseloads, multiple task increases, learning new and ever-changing regulations and guidelines, lack of control, unclear job expectations, and exacerbation of overtime. These additional stressors on top of an already taxed LTC industry resulted in increased percentages of burnout.

According to the American Medical Association, Coping with COVID-19 for Caregivers Survey administered in 2020, 49% of the individuals surveyed were experiencing burnout and the stress scores were highest among nursing assistants, medical assistants, social workers, respiratory therapists, nurses, and housekeepers. [76]

A survey of HCWs in India demonstrated that 52.8% of the respondents had pandemic-related burnout and 26.9% had work-related burnout.[77] A report in October 2022 by the Qatar Foundation World Innovation Summit for Health (WISH) in collaboration with the WHO found that burnout among HCWs during the pandemic ranged from 41% to 52% in the pooled estimates.[78] Additionally, HCW depression, anxiety, and PTSD increased during the pandemic.

Depression, Anxiety, and PTSD

Even before SARS-CoV-2, there was substantiated mental health symptomatology encompassing HCWs; researchers evaluated data from the Behavioral Risk Factor Surveillance System (BRFSS) from 2017 to 2019 and found that across the workforce, 19% of HCWs were diagnosed with depression and 41% reported insufficient sleep.[79] Depression, anxiety, and PTSD were experienced by HCWs globally during the pandemic.

Statistics

In the United States, the COVID-19 pandemic impacted the mental health of HCWs as exhibited in Figure 1.7. Based on Pulse Survey data from May 14 to 19, 2020, 28.2% of adults in the United States had symptoms of an anxiety disorder, 24.4% had symptoms of a depressive disorder, and 33.9% had symptoms of one or both disorders in the prior seven days.[80]

An analysis in Italy of moderate to extremely severe symptoms of depression and anxiety displayed 8–10% rates in the HCW population sampled.[82] Lebanon evaluated HCWs who worked directly with suspected or confirmed cases of COVID-19 and revealed that 83% of the sampled

US Percentage of HCW Mental Health Impact

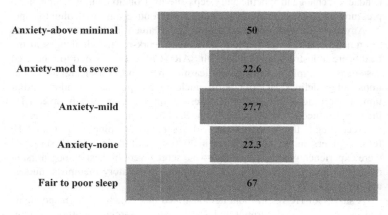

Figure 1.7 Impact of COVID-19 on US HCWs' Mental Health.[81]

Source: *Journal of Patient-Reported Outcomes.* This is a funnel diagram with a vertical axis that contains signs and symptoms of US HCW mental health impact and percentages, with a decline in sleep being the highest at 67% and no anxiety at the lowest at 22.3% during the COVID-19 pandemic.

subjects had mild to moderate levels of anxiety and 27% had moderate to high levels of anxiety.[83]

A British Medical Association survey conducted on May 14, 2020, during the pandemic, revealed that 45% of UK doctors were suffering from depression, anxiety, stress, and burnout.[84] Only nurses were assessed for depressive symptoms in China, the Philippines, the United States, Turkey, Saudi Arabia, Iran, Great Brittan, Brazil, and Canada with a combined overall rate of 22% found among this population.[85]

In Ireland, an analysis of healthcare assistants (47.5%), registered nurses (RNs) (41%), and social care workers (11.7%) employed in nursing homes was conducted to examine the differences in scores for depression and anxiety symptomatology in these populations; the results demonstrated that nurses scored the highest mean, nursing assistants were second, and social workers last.[86]

An analysis of PTSD symptoms during Wave 1 (10.73%) and Wave 2 (20.84%) of the pandemic revealed that HCWs reported higher PTSD symptomatology during Wave 2.[87] It was estimated that 21.5% of 97,333 HCWs across 21 countries experienced PTSD symptomatology during the pandemic.[88]

Morbidity and Mortality

Worldwide, HCW infections and deaths are occurring in both hospitals and LTC facilities. The pandemic impacted the medical profession on every level from nursing assistants to physicians, and demonstrates no specifics on who can be infected by SARS-CoV-2.

COVID-19 HCW Morbidity

In the United States, between June 2020 and October 2021, there were 440,044 HCWs who tested positive for COVID-19.[89] Australia reported that, as of January 12, 2023, 72,708 HCWs had been diagnosed with the SARS-CoV-2 virus in their country.[90] Since June 2021, the number of recorded COVID-19 infections in Canadian HCWs increased from 94,873 to 150,546 by January 14, 2022.[91] While the Omicron variant appeared to demonstrate lower disease severity, the largest number of new COVID-19 cases in HCWs was recorded between June 2021 and January 2022, compared with the first three waves. This had an impact on the number of staff available to provide care.[92]

In 2020, the ECDC stated that 20% of positive COVID cases in Spain were attributed to HCWs. At the same time, the Spanish Health Ministry reported that 35,295 HCWs had been infected.[93] Besides more than 35,000 health professionals infected, an EL PAÍS estimate based on available regional statistics showed that nearly 12,000 employees of senior residences and other care centers had also been infected.[94] In Italy, the second most affected European country, there were just under 18,000 infected HCWs in 2020, according to figures released by Italian Health Authorities.[95]

By May 3, 2021, there were 53,472 cases of COVID-19 in health and welfare workers confirmed by Berufsgenossenschaft für Gesundheitsdienst und Wohlfahrtspflege (BGW insurance claim) in Germany. The majority of the claims were from nurses and nurse aides (71.5%) followed by physicians (9.3%). It is suggested in this study that the number of cases of COVID-19 in this report should be doubled, as only 50% of HCWs report to BGW in Germany.[96] These statistics of HCW SARS-CoV-2 infections are similar for many countries throughout the world.

COVID-19 HCW Mortality

The WHO in 2021 estimated that the global number of HCW deaths from COVID-19 was between 80,000 and 180,000 individuals, with a median of 115,000 deaths obtained for the statistic. An analysis in Indonesia from December 2020 to July 2021 revealed that there were 1,545 HCW deaths from the SARS-CoV-2 virus.[97] Figure 1.8 illustrates HCW deaths from COVID-19 by September 2020.

COVID-19 HCW Deaths by September 2020

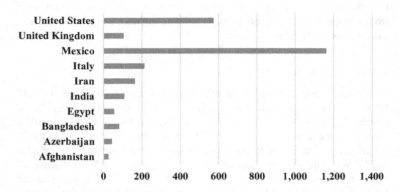

Figure 1.8 Number of HCW Deaths due to COVID-19 by September 2020.[98]

Source: *International Journal of Infectious Diseases*. This is a bar graph illustrating a horizontal axis of numbers 0–1,400 and a vertical axis of specific countries in 2020 depicting HCW COVID related deaths, with Italy being over 1,000 deaths and Afghanistan under 100.

As of January 14, 2022, at least 46 Canadian HCWs had died from COVID-19.[99] In Italy, by April 17, 2020, 117 medical doctors, 34 nurses, and 17 nurse aides had died from coronavirus.[100] An earlier 2020 Amnesty International report identified that the HCW mortality in Ecuador was 82 HCWs, in England and Wales, it was 540 HCWs, and in Brazil, 351 HCWs lost their life due to COVID-19.[101] An Amnesty International publication that was updated in March 2021 reveals HCW COVID-19 mortality as illustrated in Figure 1.9.

The global deaths and infection rates of HCWs can impact the existing workforce population by deterring individuals from pursuing the medical profession as a career choice. As new variants of the virus evolve and individuals refuse to get vaccinated, it may be more difficult to obtain herd immunity; thus, it is perceived by most epidemiologists that COVID-19 will continue to exist and will probably never obtain the eradication level of say the measles or smallpox.

In retrospect, I believe the majority of elder care facilities were not well prepared for a pandemic. The architectural design of many LTC facilities alone is an adversity to implementing COVID units and maintaining effective isolative precautions for numerous residents at one time, during an outbreak. Also, the multifactorial dynamics regarding staffing in most facilities, lack of PPE availability in many countries, and adversities in protocols globally led to successive outbreaks in many LTC facilities worldwide, which continue to occur today.

European COVID-19 HCW Mortality March 2021

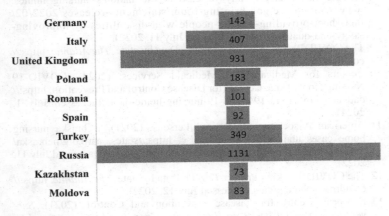

Figure 1.9 European COVID-19 HCW Mortality by March 2021.[102]

Source: Amnesty International. This is a funnel diagram containing a vertical axis that provides numbers of COVID HCW mortality in 2021, with Russia at 1,131 deaths and Kazakhstan at 73 deaths.

Notes

1 Statista. (2022). Total number of US coronavirus (COVID-19) cases as of October 5, 2022 by state. www.statista.com/ statistics/1102 807/coronavirus-covid19-cases/number/us/americans/by/state/. (accessed October 16, 2022).
2 Worldometer. (2022). COVID-19 coronavirus pandemic. www.worldom-eter.info/coronavirus. (accessed October 16, 2022).
3 The COVID Tracking Project. (2021). Data by state. *The Atlantic*. https:// covidtracking.com/data. (accessed July 12, 2022).
4 Chatterjee, Paula, et al. (2020). Characteristics and quality of US nursing homes reporting cases of coronavirus disease 2019 (COVID-19). *JAMA Network Open*. 3(7):e2016930. www.pubmed.ncbi.nlm.nih.gov/ 32725243/. (accessed July 11, 2022).
5 National Institutes of Health. (2022). How COVID-19 affects nursing homes and people with dementia. www.covid19.nih.gov/news-and-stories/ covid-19-affects-nursinghomes-dementia. (accessed July 11, 2022).
6 Centers for Medicare and Medicaid Services. (2024). COVID-19 Nursing Home Data. Centers for Disease Control and Prevention. https://data.cms. gov/covid-19/covid-19-nursing-home-data. (accessed July 1, 2024).
7 Antos, Andrew, et al. (2021). Unusually high risks of COVID-19 mortality with age-related comorbidities: An adjusted meta-analysis method to improve the risk assessment of mortality using the comorbid mortality data. *Infectious Disease Report*. 8;13(3). https://doi.org/10.3390/idr130 30065. pp. 700–711.

8 White House Briefing. (2022). Fact sheet: Protecting seniors by improving safety and quality of care in the nation's nursing homes. www.whitehouse.gov/briefing-room/statements-releases/2022/02/fact-sheet-providing-seniors-people-with-disabilities-by-improving-safety-and-quality-of-care. (accessed July 11, 2022).

9 The COVID Tracking Project. (2021). Data by state. *The Atlantic.* https://covidtracking.com/data. (accessed July 12, 2022).

10 Centers for Medicare and Medicaid Services. (2024). COVID-19 Nursing Home Data. Centers for Disease Control and Prevention. https://data.cms.gov/covid-19/covid-19-nursing-home-data. (accessed July 1, 2024).

11 American Association of Retired Persons. (2021). Nebraska nursing home cases and deaths sharply rise. https://states.aarp.org/nebraska/nebraska-nursing-home-cases-and-deaths-sharply-rising. (accessed July 11, 2022).

12 The COVID Tracking Project. (2021). Data by state. *The Atlantic.* https://covidtracking.com/data. (accessed July 12, 2022).

13 European Centre for Disease Prevention and Control. (2021). *Surveillance of COVID-19 in Long-term Care Facilities in the EU/EEA.* Stockholm: ECDC. www.ecdc.europa.eu/en/publications-data/surveillance-of-covid-19-in-long-term-care-facilities-in-the-eu-eea. (accessed July 14, 2022).

14 Anand, Janet, et al. (2021). The Covid-19 pandemic and care homes for older people in Europe-death, damage and violation of human rights. *European Journal of Social Work.* https://doi.org/10.1080/13691457.2021.1954886. (accessed July 14, 2022), pp. 804–815.

15 World Health Organization. (2020). Preventing and managing COVID-19 across long-term care services. *Policy Brief,* 25 July 2020. www.who.int/publications/i/item.who-2019-ncov-policy-brief-long-term-care-202.1. (accessed July 14, 2022).

16 European Centre for Disease Prevention and Control. (2021). *Surveillance of COVID-19 in Long-term Care Facilities in the EU/EEA November 2021.* Stockholm: ECDC. https://doi.org/10.2900/936267. p. 9.

17 Jeffay, Nathan. (2020). Why some countries suffer more from coronavirus: Israeli prof blames care homes. *The Times of Israel.* www.timesofisrael.com/why-some-countries-suffer-more-from-coronavirus-israeli-prof-blames-care-homes. (accessed July 14, 2022).

18 Vandael, Eline, et al. (2022). COVID-19 cases, hospitalizations, and deaths in Belgian homes: Results of surveillance conducted between April and December 2020. *Archives of Public Health.* 80. https://doi.org/10.1186/s13690-022-0079-6. (accessed July 16, 2022). p. 45.

19 European Centre for Disease Prevention and Control. (2021). *Surveillance of COVID-19 in Long-term Care Facilities in the EU/EEA November 2021.* Stockholm: ECDC. https://doi.org/10.2900/936267. p. 9.

20 Heneghan, C., et al. (2021). Effects of COVID-19 in care homes—a mixed methods review. *University of Oxford.* https://doi.org.10.1101/2022/04.22273903. (accessed July 18, 2022). p. 6.

21 Canadian Institute for Health. (2021). *The Impact of COVID-19 on Long Term Care in Canada: Focus on the First 6 Months.* Ottawa, ON: CIHI. www.cihi.ca/en/long-term-care-and-covid-19-the-first-6-months. (accessed July 13, 2022). p. 6.

22 Office for National Statistics. (2022). Numbers of deaths in care homes notified to the Care Quality Commission, England. www.ons.gov.uk/peoplepopulationandcommunity/birthsdeathsandmarriages/deaths/datasets/numberofdeathsincarehomesnotifiedtothecarequalitycommissionengland. (accessed July 14, 2022).

23 Rabilloud, Muriel, et al. (2022). COVID-19 outbreaks in nursing homes: A strong link with coronavirus spread in the surrounding population, France, May to July 2020. *PLoS ONE.* 17(1):e0271756. https://doi.org/10.1371/journal.pone.0261756. (accessed July 16, 2022).

24 Tarteret, Paul, and Diamantis, Sylvain. (2021). Clinical features and medical care factors associated with mortality in French nursing homes during the COVID-19 outbreak. *International Journal of Infectious Diseases.* https://doi.org/10.1016/j.ijid.2020.12.004. (accessed July 16, 2022). pp. 125–131.

25 European Centre for Disease Prevention and Control. (2021). *Surveillance of COVID-19 in Long-term Care Facilities in the EU/EEA November 2021.* Stockholm: ECDC. https://doi.org/10.2900/936267. p. 9.

26 Leao, Teresa, et al. (2021). COVID-19 transmission and case fatality in long-term care facilities during the epidemic first Wave. *Journal of American Geriatrics Society.* https://doi.org/10.111/jgs.17427. www.ncbi.nlm.nih.gov/pmc/articles/pmc8447024/. (accessed July 17, 2022). pp. 3339–3400.

27 European Centre for Disease Prevention and Control. (2021). *Surveillance of COVID-19 in Long-term Care Facilities in the EU/EEA November 2021.* Stockholm, ECDC. https://doi.org/10.2900/936267. p. 9.

28 Bethell, Jennifer et al. (2021). Social connection in long-term care homes: A scoping review of published research on the mental health impacts and potential strategies during COVID-19. *Journal of American Medical Directors Association.* 22(2). https://doi.org/10.1016.j.jamda.2020.11.025. (accessed November 6, 2022). pp. 228–232.

29 Montgomery, Anne, et al. (2020). Experiences of nursing home residents during the pandemic. *Altarum.* https:alterum.org/publications/experiences-of-nursing-home-residents-during-the-pandemic. (accessed November 5, 2022).

30 Montgomery, Anne, et al. (2020). Experiences of nursing home residents during the pandemic. *Altarum.* https:alterum.org/publications/experiences-of-nursing-home-residents-during-the-pandemic. (accessed November 5, 2022).

31 Caoimh, Ronan, et al. (2020). Psychosocial impact of COVID-19 nursing home restrictions on visitors of residents with cognitive impairment: A cross-sectional study as part of the engaging remotely in care (ERiC) project. *Frontiers in Psychiatry.* 11:1–9. https://doi.org/10.3389/psyt.2020.585373. (accessed November 6, 2022).

32 Chidambaram, Priya. (2020). *Data Note: How Might Coronavirus Affect Residents in Nursing Facilities?* Kaiser Family Foundation. https://kff. org/coronavirus-covid-19/issue-brief/data-note-how-might-coronavirus -affect-residents-in-nursing-facilities/. (accessed November 7, 2022).
33 Levere, Michael, et al. (2021). The adverse effects of the COVID-19 pandemic on nursing home resident well-being. *Journal of the American Medical Directors Association.* 22(5):e2. https://pubmed.ncbi.nlm.nih. gov/33861980/. (accessed November 7, 2022). pp. 948–954.
34 Janus, Soraya, et al. (2023). Impacts of the COVID-19 pandemic on the bereaved. *Illness, Crisis & Loss.* 0(0). https://doi.org/10.1177/1054137 3221151105. (accessed October 31, 2023).
35 Schweighart, Roxana, et al. (2021). Experiences and perspectives of nursing home residents with depressive symptoms during the COVID-19 pandemic: A qualitative study. *Zeitschrift für Gerontologie und Geriatrie.* 54. https://doi.org/10.1007/s00391-021-01926-3. (accessed November 7, 2022). pp. 353–358.
36 Schweighart, Roxana, et al. (2021). Experiences and perspectives of nursing home residents with depressive symptoms during the COVID-19 pandemic: A qualitative study. *Zeitschrift für Gerontologie und Geriatrie.* 54. https://doi.org/10.1007/s00391-021-01926-3. (accessed November 7, 2022). pp. 353–358.
37 Roest, H. G. V., et al. (2020). The impact of COVID-19 measures on well-being of older long-term care facility residents in the Netherlands. *Journal of the American Medical Directors Association.* 21(11). https:// doi.org/10.1016/j.jamda.2020.09.007. (accessed November 7, 2022). pp. 1569–1570.
38 Srifuengfung, Maytinee. (2021). Impact of the COVID-19 pandemic on older adults living in long-term care centers in Thailand, and risk factors for post-traumatic stress, depression, and Anxiety. *Journal of Affective Disorders.* 1(295). https://pubmed.ncbi.nlm.nih.gov/34488089/. (accessed November 7, 2022). pp. 353–365.
39 Roest, H. G. V., et al. (2020). The impact of COVID-19 measures on well-being of older long-term care facility residents in the Netherlands. *Journal of the American Medical Directors Association.* 21(11). https:// doi.org/10.1016/j.jamda.2020.09.007. (accessed November 7, 2022). pp. 1569–1570.
40 Sarangi, Ashish, et al. (2021). COVID-19-associated PTSD in the elderly-lessons learned for the next global pandemic. *Middle East Current Psychiatry.* 28(1). https://pubmed.ncbi.nlmnih.gov/pmc/articles/ PMC8242287/. (accessed November 7, 2022). p. 39.
41 Sarangi, Ashish, et al. (2021). COVID-19-associated PTSD in the elderly-lessons learned for the next global pandemic. *Middle East Current Psychiatry.* 28(1). https://pubmed.ncbi.nlmnih.gov/pmc/articles/ PMC8242287/. (accessed November 7, 2022). p. 39.
42 Sarangi, Ashish, et al. (2021). COVID-19-associated PTSD in the elderly-lessons learned for the next global pandemic. *Middle East Current Psychiatry.* 28(1). https://pubmed.ncbi.nlmnih.gov/pmc/articles/ PMC8242287/. (accessed November 7, 2022). p. 39.

43 Sarangi, Ashish, et al. (2021). COVID-19-associated PTSD in the elderly-lessons learned for the next global pandemic. *Middle East Current Psychiatry.* 28(1). https://pubmed.ncbi.nlmnih.gov/pmc/articles/PMC8242287/. (accessed November 7, 2022). p. 39.
44 Sarangi, Ashish, et al. (2021). COVID-19-associated PTSD in the elderly-lessons learned for the next global pandemic. *Middle East Current Psychiatry.* 28(1). https://pubmed.ncbi.nlmnih.gov/pmc/articles/PMC8242287/. (accessed November 7, 2022). p. 39.
45 Kerns, William, et al. (2022). *Management of Dementia Related Behaviors During COVID: A Virginia Nursing Home Clinician Survey, November 2021.* The Larry A. Green Center. www.green-center.org/blog/management-of-dementia-related-behaviors-during-covid-a-virginia-nursing-home-clinician-survey-november-2021. (accessed November 21, 2022).
46 Benzinger, Petra, et al. (2023). Consequences of contact restrictions for long-term care residents during the first months of COVID-19 pandemic: A scoping review. *European Journal of Ageing.* 20(39). https://doi.org/10.1007/s10433-023-00787-6. (accessed October 31, 2023).
47 Hoel, Viktoria, et al. (2022). Social health among German Nursing home residents with dementia during the COVID-19 pandemic, and the role of technology to promote social participation. *International Journal of Environmental Research and Public Health.* 19(4). https://doi.org/10.3390/ijerph19041956. (accessed November 20, 2022). p. 956.
48 Simonetti, Alessio, et al. (2020). Neuropsychiatric symptoms in elderly with dementia during COVID-19 pandemic: Definition, treatment, and future directions. *Frontiers in Psychiatry.* 11. https://pubmed.ncbi.nlm.nih.gov/33132939/. (accessed November 21, 2022). p. 579842.
49 Kippenberg, Inge, et al. (2022). Stimuli changes and challenging behavior in nursing homes during the COVID-19 pandemic. *BMC Geriatrics.* 22. https://doi.org/10.1186/s12887-022-02824-y. (accessed November 21, 2022). p. 142.
50 Scerri, Anthony, PhD, et al. (2022). Nurses' experiences of caring for long-term care residents with dementia during the COVID-18 pandemic. *Gerontology and Geriatric Medicine.* 8. https://doi.org/23337214221077793. https://pubmed.ncbi.nlm.nih.gov/35261915/. (accessed November 21, 2022).
51 Martinchek, Michelle, et al. (2020). Weight loss in COVID-19 positive nursing home residents. *Journal of the American Medical Directors Association.* 22(2). https://pubmed.ncbi.nlm.nih.gov/33352194. (accessed November 9, 2022). pp. 257–259.
52 Danilovich, Margaret, et al. (2020). Nursing home resident weight loss during coronavirus disease 2019 restrictions. *Journal of the American Medical Directors Association.* 21(11). https://pubmed.ncbi.nlm.nih.gov/33138939. (accessed November 9, 2022). pp. 1568–1569.
53 Levere, Michael, et al. (2021). The adverse effects of COVID-19 pandemic on nursing home resident well-being. *Journal of the American Medical Directors Association.* 22(5). https://pubmed.ncbi.nlm.nih.gov/33861980/. pp. 948–954.

54 Sanchez, M. J., et al. (2021). Weight loss in nursing home older adults during the first COVID-19 pandemic wave: Viral infection or disruption of nutritional care organization? LB-102. *Clinical Nutrition ESPN.* 46. www.ncbi.nlm.nih.gov/pmc/articles/PMC8629552/. (accessed October 31, 2023). p. 784.

55 Perez-Rodriguez, Patricia. (2021). Functional, cognitive, and nutritional decline in 435 elderly nursing home residents after the first wave of the COVID-19 pandemic. *European Geriatric Medicine.* 12. https://doi.org/10.1007/s41999-021-00534-1. (accessed November 13, 2022). pp. 1137–1145.

56 Perez-Rodriguez, Patricia. (2021). Functional, cognitive. And nutritional decline in 435 elderly nursing home residents after the first wave of the COVID-19 pandemic. *European Geriatric Medicine.* 12. https://doi.org/10.1007/s41999-021-00534-1. (accessed November 13, 2022). pp. 1137–1145.

57 Bastami, Masoumeh, and Azadi, Arman. (2020). Effects of a multicomponent program on fall incidence, fear of falling, and quality of life among older adult nursing home residents. *Annals of Geriatric Medicine and Research.* 24(4). www.ncbi.nlm.nih.gov/pmc/articles/PMC7781964. (accessed November 15, 2022). pp. 252–258.

58 Keenan, John. (2021). *COVID-19's Effect on Common Nursing Home Injuries.* University of Nebraska Medical Center. https://unmc.edu/newsroom/2021/08/20/covid-19s-effect-on-common-nursing-home-injuries/. (accessed November 15, 2022).

59 Lambardo, Flavia, et al. (2020). Adverse events in Italian nursing homes during the COVID-19 epidemic: A national survey. *Frontiers in Psychiatry.* 11:1–9. https://doi.org/10.3389/psyt.2020.578465. (accessed November 15, 2022).

60 Health Quality Ontario. (2021). System performance: Long-term care home residents who fell. www.hqontario.ca/System-Performance/Long-Term-Care-Home-Performance/Falls. (accessed November 15, 2022).

61 Keenan, John. (2021). *COVID-19's Effect on Common Nursing Home Injuries.* University of Nebraska Medical Center. https://unmc.edu/newsroom/2021/08/20/covid-19s-effect-on-common-nursing-home-injuries/. (accessed November 15, 2022).

62 Bedsore Law. (2022). 10 nursing home stats and why they matter. www.bedsore.law/news/nursing-home-stats/. (accessed November 23, 2022).

63 Furtado, Katia, et al. (2023). The relationship between nursing practice environment and pressure ulcer care quality in Portugal's long-term care units. *Healthcare.* 11(12). https://doi.org/10.3390/healthcare11121751. (accessed October 31, 2023). p. 1751

64 Illinois Department of Public Health. (2022). Nursing home violations for first quarter of 2022. https://dph.illinois.gov/resource-center/news/2022/june/nursing-home-violations-for-first-quarter-of-2022-.html. (accessed November 24, 2022).

65 Illinois Department of Public Health. (2022). Nursing home violations for first quarter of 2022. https://dph.illinois.gov/resource-center/news/2022/

june/nursing-home-violations-for-first-quarter-of-2022-.html. (accessed November 24, 2022).
66 Incredible Health. (2022). Study: 34% of nurses plan to leave their current role by the end of 2022. www.incrediblehealth.com/wp-content/uploads/2022/03/IH-COVID-19–2022-Summary-1.pdf. (accessed October 31, 2023).
67 Xu, Huiwen, et al. (2020). Shortages of staff in nursing homes during the COVID-10 pandemic: What are driving factors? *Journal of the American Medical Directors Association.* 21(10). www.pubmed.ncbi.nlm.nih.gov/32981663/. pp. 1371–1377.
68 International Council of Nurses. (2020). The global nursing shortage and nurse retention. www.icn.ch/sites/default/files/inline-files/ICN%20Policy%20Brief_Nurse%20Shortage%20and%20Retention.pdf. (accessed January 9, 2023).
69 International Council of Nurses. (2020). The global nursing shortage and nurse retention. www.icn.ch/sites/default/files/inline-files/ICN%20Policy%20Brief_Nurse%20Shortage%20and%20Retention.pdf. (accessed January 9, 2023).
70 International Council of Nurses. (2020). The global nursing shortage and nurse retention. www.icn.ch/sites/default/files/inline-files/ICN%20Policy%20Brief_Nurse%20Shortage%20and%20Retention.pdf. (accessed January 9, 2023).
71 International Council of Nurses. (2020). The global nursing shortage and nurse retention. www.icn.ch/sites/default/files/inline-files/ICN%20Policy%20Brief_Nurse%20Shortage%20and%20Retention.pdf. (accessed January 9, 2023).
72 International Council of Nurses. (2020). The global nursing shortage and nurse retention. www.icn.ch/sites/default/files/inline-files/ICN%20Policy%20Brief_Nurse%20Shortage%20and%20Retention.pdf. (accessed January 9, 2023).
73 International Council of Nurses. (2020). The global nursing shortage and nurse retention. www.icn.ch/sites/default/files/inline-files/ICN%20Policy%20Brief_Nurse%20Shortage%20and%20Retention.pdf. (accessed January 9, 2023).
74 Schwartz, Emma. (2022). The global health care worker shortage: 10 numbers to note. *Project Hope.* www.projecthope.org/the-global-health-worker-shortage-10-numbers-to-note/04/2022/. (accessed January 9, 2023).
75 Schwartz, Emma. (2022). The global health care worker shortage: 10 numbers to note. *Project Hope.* www.projecthope.org/the-global-health-worker-shortage-10-numbers-to-note/04/2022/. (accessed January 9, 2023).
76 Mental Health America. (2022). The mental health of healthcare workers in COVID-19. https://mhanational.org/mental-health-healthcare-workers-covid-19. (accessed January 6, 2023).
77 Khasne, Ruchira. (2020). Burnout among healthcare workers during COVID-19 pandemic in India: Results of a questionnaire-based survey.

Indian Journal of Critical Care Medicine. 24(8). www.ncbi.nlm.gov/pmc/articles/PMC7519601/. (accessed January 6, 2023). pp. 664–671.

78 World Health Organization. (2022). World failing in "our duty of care" to protect mental health and well-being of health and care workers finds report on impact of COVID-19. www.who.int/item/05-10-2022-world-failing-in-our-duty-of-care-to-protect-mental-health-and-wellbeing-of-health-and-care-workers-finds-report-on-impact-of-covid-19. (accessed January 6, 2023).

79 Silver, Sharon, et al. (2022). *Pre-pandemic Mental Health and Well-being of Healthcare Workers.* Centers for Disease Control and Prevention. https://blogs.cdc.gov/niosh-science-blog/2022/08/29/hcw-mental-health-prepandemic/. (accessed January 10, 2023).

80 National Center for Health Statistics. (2020). Early release of selected mental health estimates based on data from the January – June 2019 national health interview survey. www.cdc.gov/nchs/data/nhis/earlyrelease/ERmentalhealth-508.pdf. (accessed October 31, 2023).

81 Biber, Joshua. (2022). Mental health impact on healthcare workers due to COVID-19 pandemic: A U.S. cross-sectional study. *Journal of Patient-Reported Outcomes.* 6. https://doi.org/10.1186/s41687-022-00467-6. (accessed January 10, 2023). p. 63.

82 Lenzo, Vittorio. (2021). Depression, anxiety, and stress among healthcare workers during COVID-19 outbreaks and relationships with expressive flexibility and context sensibility. *Frontiers in Psychology.* 12:1–9. https://doi.org/10.3389.psyg.2021.623933. (accessed January 10, 2023).

83 Sakr, C. J., et al. (2022). Anxiety among Healthcare Workers during COVID-19 Pandemic in Lebanon: The Importance of the Work Environment and Personal Resilience. *Dove Medical Press.* www.dovepress.com/anxiety-among-healthcare-workers-during-covid-19-pandemic-in-lebanon-t-peer-reviewed-fulltext-article-PRBM. (accessed January 10, 2023). pp. 811–821.

84 De Kock, Johannes, et al. (2021). A rapid review of the impact of COVID-19 on the mental health of healthcare workers: implications for supporting psychological well-being. *BMC Public Health.* 21(104). https://doi.org/10.1186/s12889-020-10070-3. (accessed January 10, 2023).

85 Slusarska, Barbaram, et al. (2022). Prevalence of depression and anxiety in nurses during the first eleven months of the COVID-19 pandemic: A systematic review and meta-analysis. *International Journal of Environmental Research and Public Health.* 19(3). https://pub.med.ncbi.nlm.nih.gov/35162183/. (accessed January 10, 2023). p. 1154.

86 Hughes, Megan. (2022). Stress, anxiety, and depression among nursing home healthcare workers during a pandemic. https://norma.ncirl.ie/5653/1/me. (accessed January 10, 2023).

87 Ouyang, Hui, et al. (2022). The increase of PTSD in front-line health care workers during COVID-19 pandemic and the mediating role of risk perception: One-year follow-up study. *Translational Psychiatry.* 12(180). https://doi.org/10.1038/s41398-022001953-7. (accessed January 10, 2023).

88 Li, Yufei, et al. (2021). Prevalence of depression, anxiety, and post-traumatic stress disorder in health care workers during COVID-19 pandemic: A systematic review and meta-analysis. *PLOS ONE.* 16(3). https://doi.org/10.1371/journal.pone.0246454. (accessed January 10, 2023). p. e0246454.

89 Lin, S., et al. (2022). COVID-19 symptoms and deaths among healthcare workers, United States. *Emerging Infectious Diseases, CDC.* 28(8). https://doi.org/10.3201/eid2808.212200. (accessed January 16, 2023). pp. 1624–1641.

90 Australian Department of Health and Aged Care. (2023). Coronavirus (COVID-19) case numbers and statistics. https://www.health.gov.au/sites/default/files/2023-01/covid-19-outbreaks-in-australian-residential-aged-care-facilities-13-january-2023_0.pdf. (accessed January 16, 2023).

91 Canadian Institute of Health Information. (2022). COVID-19 cases and deaths in health care workers in Canada. www.cihi.ca/en/covid-19-cases-and-deaths-in-health-care-workers-in-canada. (accessed January 16, 2023).

92 Canadian Institute of Health Information. (2022). COVID-19 cases and deaths in health care workers in Canada. www.cihi.ca/en/covid-19-cases-and-deaths-in-health-care-workers-in-canada. (accessed January 16, 2023).

93 Guell, Oriol. (2020). Spain ranks first for COVID-19 infections among healthcare workers. *El Pais.* https://english.elpais.com/spanish_news/2020-04-25/spain-ranks-first-for-covid-19-infections-among-healthcare-workers.html. (accessed January 16, 2023).

94 Guell, Oriol. (2020). Spain ranks first for COVID-19 infections among health-care workers. *El Pais.* https://english.elpais.com/spanish_news/2020-04-25/spain-ranks-first-for-covid-19-infections-among-healthcare-workers.html. (accessed January 16, 2023).

95 Guell, Oriol. (2020). Spain ranks first for COVID-19 infections among healthcare workers. *El Pais.* https://english.elpais.com/spanish_news/2020-04-25/spain-ranks-first-for-covid-19-infections-among-healthcare-workers.html. (accessed January 16, 2023).

96 Nienhaus, Albert. (2021). COVID-19 among health workers in Germany-An update. *International Journal of Environmental Research and Public Health.* 18(17). www.ncbi.nlm.nih.gov/pmc/articles/PMC8431697/. (accessed January 17, 2023). p. 9185.

97 Ekawati, L. L., et al. (2022). Mortality among healthcare workers in Indonesia during 18 months of COVID-19. *PLOS Global Public Health.* 2(12). https://doi.org/10.1371/journal.pgph.0000893. (accessed January 16, 2023). p. e0000893.

98 Erdem, Hakan, and Lucey, Daniel. (2020). Healthcare worker infections and deaths due to COVID-19: A survey of 37 nations and a call for WHO to post national data on their website. *International Journal of Infectious Diseases.* 102:239–241. https://doi.org/10.1016/j.isid.2020.10.064. (accessed January 16, 2023).

99   Canadian Institute of Health Information. (2022). COVID-19 cases and deaths in health care workers in Canada. www.cihi.ca/en/covid-19-cases-and-deaths-in-health-care-workers-in-canada. (accessed January 16, 2023).

100 Lapolla, Pierfrancesco, et al. (2020). Deaths from COVID-19 in healthcare workers in Italy-what can we learn? *Infection Control & Hospital Epidemiology.* www.cambridge.org/core/journals/infection-control-and-hospital-epidemiology/article/deaths-from-covid19-in-healthcare-workers-in-italywhat-can-we-learn/BDA8BA987868E2B86B50F0D070496827. (accessed January 18, 2023). pp. 1, 2.

101 Amnesty International. (2020). UK among highest COVID-19 health worker deaths in the world. www.amnesty.org.uk/press-releases/uk-among-highest-covid-19-health-worker-deaths-world. (accessed January 18, 2023).

102 European Public Service Union. (2021). The COVID-19 death toll of health and care workers continue to rise. www.epsu.org/sites/default/files/article/files/AMNESTY%20INTERNATIONAL   HEALTH%20WORKERS-%20DEATH%20DUE%20TO%20COVID%2019.pdf. (accessed January 18, 2023).

2 Operators

Corporations, Government, and Private Sector

Business adversities impacting for-profit, non-profit, and governmental owned nursing homes related to the coronavirus pandemic elicited federal/ governmental interventions globally to assist in sustaining the industry. LTC facility closures are still occurring globally due to rising costs, increased regulatory pressures, decreased staffing, and insufficient state subsidies for care. An article published in *Bloomberg Law* written by Tony Pugh, "Bankruptcies, Closures Loom for Nursing Homes Beset by Pandemic," reported:

> More than 120 nursing homes have already closed in 2020 and "another 150 or so are at risk for closing in the next few months," said Mark Parkinson, president and CEO of the American Health Care Association, which represents more than 14,000 nursing homes and long-term care facilities.[1]

The Centers for Medicare & Medicaid Services (CMS) announced that 129 nursing homes closed nationally in 2022.[2] Figure 2.1 depicts the number of facilities closed in some specific US states. Yet, another report disclosed that as of April 2022, 327 nursing homes in the United States had closed during the pandemic, affecting the displacement of 12,775 nursing home residents.[3] In addition, approximately 60% of American nursing homes surveyed reported that they were operating at a financial loss in 2022.[4] One administrative staff member stated:

> at the worst we had ten empty beds which probably (in a) 62 bed home doesn't sound like much but you are talking about a lot of money every month and if we were private, we might have decided to cut our losses and close or sell up as a number of homes around here have.[5]

In an American Health Care Association and National Center for Assisted Living Report, released in August 2023, it is revealed that, since 2020, nearly 600 nursing homes have closed. And, in 2023, only three new nursing homes

DOI: 10.4324/9781003466192-4

2022 Nursing Home Closures in the United States

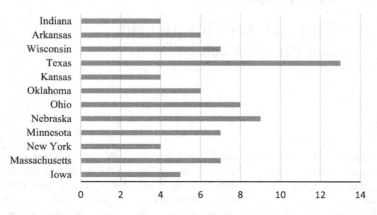

Figure 2.1 Nursing Home Closures in the United States by 2022.[6]

Source: Becker's Hospital Review. This bar graph illustrates a vertical axis of specific US states and a horizontal axis of numbers 0–14, showing the number of nursing home closures by 2022, with Texas having the most closures at over 12 facilities, and Indiana, New York, and Kansas having the least demonstrating four or less facilities that closed.

opened—a major drop from the average of 64 new nursing homes per year from 2020 to 2022.[7]

Nursing Homes Ireland (NHI) reported that 17 nursing homes had closed by April 2022, with a loss of approximately 500 jobs.[8] Some news articles in Ontario, Canada, disclosed that nursing homes were closing in 2022, leaving staff members without a job and the hospital working to rehome the seniors. In 2021, newspapers released that one of the UK's largest care home companies, HC-One would sell many of its facilities to focus on more specialized care and it would be closing four homes. And, in 2020, Italy was reporting unless they were provided with assistance regarding costs that bankruptcy would have to be filed regarding a company that managed 30 care homes in the region around Cremona.[9]

Assistance to Nursing Homes in the United States

In America, the support furnished to the LTC industry included the Provider Relief Fund, from the Coronavirus Aid, Relief, and Economic Security (CARES) Act established in March 2020 that included a sum of about $21 billion paid out; the Paycheck Protection Program which was $5.7 billion to nursing homes; and the Medicare accelerated payment funds. The

Department of Health and Human Services (HHS) distributed the CARES Act to corporate and private sector owners in three phases:

1. Phase 1: Announced in May 2020, all certified skilled nursing home facilities (SNFs) with six or more certified beds were eligible for $50,000 per facility, in addition to $2,500 per bed. More than 13,000 SNFs received a total of $4.9 billion.
2. Phase 2: Announced in July 2020, $5 billion would be utilized to enhance nursing home response to COVID-19 and build nursing home skills. This monetary amount was distributed in two phases—$2.5 billion in August 2020 and $2 billion in Phase 3.
3. Phase 3: Announced in September 2020, the $2 billion would be dispersed based on performance-based incentive payments to nursing home facilities, determined by specific infection and death rates related to COVID-19.[10]

The monetary amounts provided to nursing homes were partially utilized on increased PPE and staffing expenditures.

PPE Expenditures

Most nursing homes were reporting that they were spending their annual PPE budget in just one month during the pandemic. Presbyterian Homes and Services estimated that the average 72-bed nursing home was spending an additional $2,265 per day on PPE during the pandemic.[11] Another study revealed that the nursing home industry spent approximately $20 billion on PPE and staffing in 2020 alone.[12] The Federal Emergency Management Agency (FEMA) sent a 14-day supply of PPE to 15,000 nursing homes in May 2020, which assisted with cost factors in these facilities for a month.[13]

Staffing Expenditures

Staffing cost expenditures increased partly due to the increased utilization of contract (agency) staff. One analysis reported that nursing homes used 24% more contract staff in 2020 than in 2019, including RNs, licensed practical nurses, and certified nursing assistants.[14]

SmartLinx, a workforce management solutions company, revealed that the number of shifts allocated to agency staff was up 154%, from 145,423 in 2019 to 370,740 in 2020.[15] Agency salaries for nursing home staff generally are higher, and the average hourly wages in the United States are:

• RN $45.21/hour
• LPN 27.68/hour
• CNA 17.56/hour

Some states made changes to their staffing requirements after the onset of COVID-19; Arkansas, Connecticut, Massachusetts, New York, and Rhode Island adopted permanent increases to minimum staffing requirements and Georgia adopted a permanent decrease.[16] The American Health Care Association and National Center for Assisted Living (AHCS/NCAL) estimate, that within a two-year period (2020–2021), the LTC industry lost $94 billion, due to increased costs to fight the pandemic and declining revenues.[17]

Staffing Shortages Contributed to Closures

As stated previously, the COVID-19 pandemic exacerbated staffing problems. According to the Bureau of Labor Statistics, from February 2020 to November 2021, the number of workers in nursing homes and other care facilities dropped by 410,000 nationally. And, staffing has only rebounded by about 103,000 (2023) since then.[18]

A recent "State of the Nursing Home Industry Survey" conducted by the American Healthcare Association and reported on in early 2023 identified that 86% of US nursing homes were experiencing moderate to severe staffing shortages, 96% were struggling to hire staff, and 78% had hired agency staff.[19]

In an attempt to mitigate staffing adversities in LTC during the pandemic, many states, corporations, and facilities instituted hazard pay, bonuses, and/or permanently increased wages. At least four states (i.e., Colorado, Illinois, Massachusetts, and North Carolina) adopted laws or regulations that required increases in nursing home staff wages, and three states (i.e., Mississippi, North Carolina, Ohio) adopted temporary increases in wages and/or additional one-time bonuses.[20]

The Public Health Institute (PHI) published a whitepaper detailing hazard pay and sick leave policies in nursing homes across the United States between March 2020 and August 2021–24 states and the District of Columbia supported direct care givers with hazard pay and/or sick leave; just 10 states implemented both.[21] A survey conducted by Kaiser Family Foundation in 2021 revealed that 58% of nursing home employees felt employers fell short of providing additional compensation during the pandemic, even with federal assistance being provided to offset hardship.[22]

In October 2023, it was identified that nursing homes lost more workers than other healthcare sectors; 250,000 jobs were lost in nursing homes in the United States, translating to about 15% of the workforce. While many other sectors have rebounded after the pandemic, projections estimate that nursing homes will not hit pre-pandemic staffing levels until 2026.[23] Globally, the nursing home industry in many other countries exhibited similar economic hardships.

Assistance to Nursing Homes in Other Countries

In April 2020, the Ministry of Health in Ireland enacted the Temporary Assistance Scheme; the core concept of the scheme is that the State would provide additional funding to those nursing homes that require it, to contribute toward costs associated with SARS-CoV-2 preparedness, mitigation, and outbreak management. The scheme consisted of two components: (a) a support payment per month based on the number of residents in a facility and (b) enhanced assistance in the event of a nursing home actively managing an outbreak, consisting of the Outbreak Assistance Scheme that paid €1,800 per resident, subject to a maximum of €33,000 to contribute toward costs associated with COVID-19 in nursing homes.[24]

United Kingdom

The UK government in March 2020 announced a funding of €1.6 billion for local governments and an additional €1.3 billion to go to the NHS and Social Care for discharge support. Additionally, in April 2020, it was announced that a further €1.6 billion was to be provided for Local Government to assist financially during the pandemic, and the country's detailed Adult Social Care Action Plan was released.

Then in May 2020, the government announced a care homes support package in the United Kingdom backed by a €600 million adult social care infection control fund.[25] Another announcement from the Department of Health and Social Care in May 2022 stated that providers would receive an additional €87 million for nursing care during the pandemic in 2021 and 2022, and an additional 11.5% increase in funding for 2022 and 2023.[26] Figure 2.2 illustrates countries that contributed to the financial support of HCWs during the pandemic.

Canada

The Canadian Government helped nursing homes in provinces and territories during the pandemic by providing funding of over $39 million through the Canadian Red Cross.[27] In addition, Canada implemented a government program of $10 million a month allocated to nursing homes for staff salaries in support of a directive for employees to only work in one facility.[28] Additionally, a Safe LTC fund of $1 billion was established to assist nursing homes in Canada.[29]

Australia

Australian Government assistance entailed the allocation of $52.9 million over a two-year period (2019–2021) through the Aged Care Support Program to assist nursing homes that had two components: a base finding allocation of $20,000 and $2,000 for each operational facility.[31] In 2021 and 2022, the program was extended until 2023, and the grant money allocated for nursing homes increased to $191.5 million.[32]

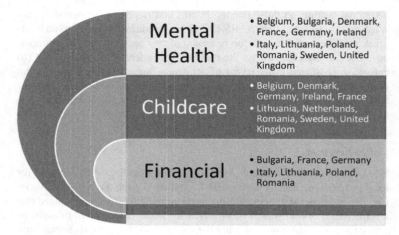

Figure 2.2 Additional Financial Support to HCWs During the Pandemic.[30]

Source: *Eurohealth.* This design art is a circular diagram with three rectangular boxes depicting countries that provided financial support, mental health assistance, and childcare support to HCWs during the pandemic; France, Germany, Lithuania, Norway, and the United Kingdom assisted with childcare expenditures.

PPE Assistance

One study surveyed OECD countries on PPE assistance provided by governments. Most of the 38 OECD members that received PPE assistance were from Europe, including Austria, Belgium, Czech Republic, Denmark, Estonia, Finland, France, Germany, Greece, Hungary, Iceland, Ireland, Italy, Latvia, Lithuania, Luxembourg, Netherlands, Norway, Poland, Portugal, Slovak Republic, Slovenia, Spain, Sweden, Switzerland, and the United Kingdom.

Korea developed a strategy to avoid shortages of PPE early on in the pandemic (March 2020), by establishing a group to manage supplies and IT systems to distribute 5.46 million public masks for 770,000 employees via LTC providers.[33] Among the surveyed countries, only in Colombia and the Czech Republic, did workers contribute to the purchase of PPE.[34] In Japan, each LTC facility paid for their own PPE, but when there was an increase in the utilization of PPE, the national or sub-national government provided PPE for free.[35]

The England Action Plan addressed PPE shortages, stating as of April 6, 2020, we will be providing essential PPE supplies to 58,000 different providers including care homes.[36] In Australia, the National Medical Stockpile (NMS) was a resource for nursing homes for emergency situations related to PPE[37]; PPE stockpiles will be discussed in the next chapter. Lack of adequate staffing to handle the pandemic also occurred globally.

Mitigation for Staffing Shortages

In an OECD survey, around 90% of the countries prepared rapid response teams at either the national or subnational level to counteract staffing shortages. In Italy, home care workers were deployed into nursing homes during staffing shortages. Austria moved LTC employees from areas of non-transmission to areas with outbreaks in need of additional staff. And, in at least four countries (i.e., Canada, Czech Republic, Estonia, and Germany), the army deployed personnel to facilities in need.[38] In addition, Portugal hastened the accreditation of foreign diplomas; Luxembourg signed short-term contracts with foreign workers, and in Australia, international students were temporarily allowed to work.[39]

Australia through the Aged Care Support Program for care homes provided a temporary surge workforce and emergency response teams for staff illnesses and outbreaks. There was also implementation of the Aged Care Worker COVID-19 leave payment grant for employees who tested positive for coronavirus with no personal leave entitlements.[40]

Approximately, 40% of the OECD countries surveyed provided one-off bonuses to reward LTC workers for their exceptional efforts. And, four countries improved care worker wages permanently at the start of the pandemic: Czech Republic Germany, France, and Korea.[41] Staffing ratios were also assessed:

- Japan, Lithuania, the Netherlands, and Slovenia introduced guidelines for staffing ratios.
- Ontario, Canada, announced a commitment to increase direct care hours by four hours/resident by 2024/2025.
- Colombia is adopting a regulation to set a staffing ratio in LTC of one staff member to every 12 patients.
- Finland, under the Older Person's Care Act, stated that they would increase their staffing ratios from 0.5 to 0.7 by 2023.[42]

Nursing Home Liability

As of June 2021 in the United States, 38 states had granted immunity to nursing homes to combat COVID-19 liabilities. Ten states issued executive orders and 28 states passed legislature that provided some form of immunity for LTC facilities, related to SARS-CoV-2. These processes were executed to protect facilities from lawsuits being instigated, despite not having control of viral transmissions. California and Florida both experienced a high number of COVID-19-related lawsuits, due to not providing immunity for their LTC facilities.

Dr. R. Tamara Konetzka of the University of Chicago stated,

multiple rigorous studies have found standard quality metrics do not have a meaningful association with COVID-19 outcomes for nursing homes, even prior infection control citations were not associated with pandemic outcomes. And, more than 99% of nursing homes in the nation have had at least one coronavirus case, and more than 80% have had at least one death, this is not a bad-apples problem.[43]

Both AARP and the Medicaid Center for Public Representation opposed immunity for the LTC industry, stating that immunity was not necessary, placed residents at risk, and harmed patients. In Nebraska, LB139 removes liability, as long as there is compliance with federal mandates in a facility, protecting both HCWs and nursing homes, yet AARP does not feel employees need protection.

Ontario, Canada, implemented statutory protection from COVID-19 liability in November 2020 with Bill 218, *Supporting Ontario's Recovery and Municipal Elections Act, 2020*. It protects both individuals and corporations, and was retroactive back to March 2020, but does not apply in cases of gross negligence.[44] Worldwide, there have been multiple lawsuits filed in relation to SARS-CoV-2, even with some countries having additional immunity protections instituted.

Actual COVID Lawsuit Cases

The Public Readiness and Emergency Preparedness Act (PREP Act), an act established by Congress in 2005, that provides immunity from liability from some legal claims, with the exception of willful misconduct, is being utilized in the US states that did not provide additional protections. However, wrongful death lawsuits (personal injury) persist as one of the avenues being utilized for litigation related to COVID and are usually based on substandard precautionary measures or care, classified as gross negligence.

> In the case of Garcia v. Welltower OpCo Group, LLC, the California federal court found the PREP Act provided immunity in a suit alleging elder abuse and neglect, wrongful death, and intentional infliction of emotional distress.[45]

A nursing home in Glendale, California, operated by Glenhaven Healthcare had a resident die from COVID-19 in 2020, and the family proceeded with litigation accusing the facility of elder abuse, willful misconduct, negligence, and wrongful death. In November 2022, the US Supreme Court declined to hear the operator's bid to avoid a lawsuit, eradicating the possibility of moving the case into federal court to gain immunity from litigation and allowing the family to proceed with a lawsuit in a California state court.[46] Many nursing homes are facing lawsuits in New Jersey; one example is the Woodland Behavioral Health and Nursing Center, and its sister site, Limecrest Subacute and Rehabilitation Center, a total of 16 families are suing the facilities for COVID-19-related deaths that occurred in the spring of 2020, stating that the deaths were preventable.[47]

In another New Jersey case, the families of two women who died in nursing homes from COVID-19 are suing the state citing that the Governor and Health Commissioner violated the residents' civil rights, stating the state ignored repeated warnings in the first weeks of the pandemic, and its controversial approaches to containing COVID in LTC facilities was deadly. The basis of the lawsuit is liability under the "state-created danger doctrine" that enables citizens to pursue remedies when the government—responsible for protecting the public—instead takes actions that endanger it. In December 2022, the state agreed to pay $52.9 million to relatives of 119 people who lived in state-run veteran's homes who died of COVID-19.[48]

Brooklyn, New York state officials are also facing lawsuits in relation to exhibiting "deliberate indifference" toward nursing home residents and causing 15,000 avoidable COVID-19 deaths.[49]

A lawsuit was filed against Brighton Rehabilitation and Wellness Center in Pennsylvania on behalf of five residents and family members of ten residents who died from COVID-19, stating that the facility was chronically understaffed, failed to separate infected residents from non-infected residents, allowed employees to work when infected, and provided inaccurate information to families and health officials.[50]

Life Care Center in Kirkland, Washington, had a lawsuit filed against them in 2020, by a family member of a resident who died after being diagnosed with COVID, alleging fraud and wrongful death stating the nursing home, "lacked a clear plan of action leading to a systemic failure," further elaborating that the facility had an outbreak, did not quarantine residents, but instead held a Mardi Gras party.[51]

The Justice Department announced on June 30, 2022, that MorseLife Nursing Home Health System Inc. agreed to pay the United States $1.75 million to resolve potential liability under False Claims Act for facilitating COVID-19 vaccinations for hundreds of individuals ineligible to participate in the CDC's Pharmacy Partnership for Long-Term Care Program, a program specifically designed to vaccinate LTC facility residents and staff when doses of COVID-19 vaccine were limited in supply at the beginning of the vaccination program.[52]

Canada

Ontario, Canada, is experiencing class-action lawsuits related to COVID, stating that the province was "grossly negligent" in failing to prevent waves of LTC deaths in the early stages of the pandemic. A judge ruled that families of nursing home victims can sue the minister of LTC, citing the plaintiffs' contention that the government showed bad faith and an acute degree of negligence.[53]

Ireland

Dealgan House Nursing Home in Dundalk, Ireland, has a wrongful death legal action pending related to a 2020 resident COVID death.[54] Also, CareChoice Ballynoe in Co Cork, Ireland, is being sued by a family member for the 2021 death of his wife related to COVID, stating that "we are forced to go the legal route to get answers."[55] It is reported that up to 30 families in Ireland are suing care homes and the Health Service Executive (HSE) claiming that nursing homes failed to follow adequate measures to protect vulnerable residents from SARS-CoV-2.

England

A high court judgment related to COVID-19 deaths in nursing homes in England (Hampshire and Oxfordshire) found that policies on admissions to nursing homes that had been instituted by the Secretary of State for Health and Social Care and Public Health England during the pandemic were irrational. The court examined the history of policy development with emphasis on symptomatic and pre-symptomatic transmission and infection, discharge from hospitals, guidance on arrangements to be adopted by care homes, testing, and PPE.[56]

Spain

In 2020, Spain's Supreme Court ordered an investigation into the deaths of elderly people in nursing homes and lack of PPE. The high court also asked the lower courts to assess the possible misuse of public funds to purchase flawed or fraudulent equipment to fight the pandemic.

However, it rejected about 50 cases that specifically targeted the government for its management of the pandemic, arguing that the complaints were not detailed enough to charge any high-ranking officials.[57]

The many adversities impacting the LTC industry related to SARS-CoV-2 provide insight into the consequences faced by operators of nursing homes. Gerontological patient complications related to the aging process, such as a compromised immune system and comorbidities, do not become a factor in wrongful death litigation cases. Staffing problems are blamed on the owners of nursing homes, even when the market for direct care staff and healthcare professionals worldwide has dramatically decreased. And, the inability to procure PPE, due to market shortages, becomes the nursing home operator's fault too.

The elder care industry needs to be reformed, including assistance with restructuring of its buildings, staffing, IPC standards, improved monetary resources for in-home care, and devising alternate mitigation strategies that are pandemic-focused. The remainder of the chapters will focus on specific protocols and policies that have been and can be implemented in LTC to improve gerontological healthcare provisions.

Notes

1 Pugh, Tony. (2020). Bankruptcies, closures loom for nursing homes beset by pandemic. *Bloomberg Law.* https://news.bloomberglaw.com/ health-law-and-business/bankruptcies-closures-loom-for-nursing-homes-beset-by-pandemic. (accessed March 28, 2023).
2 Leys, Tony. (2023). *Wave of Rural Nursing Home Closures Grows Amid Staff Crunch.* Kaiser Family Foundation. https://khn.org/news/article/ wave-of-rural-nursing-home-closures-grows-amid-staffing-crunch/. (accessed March 28, 2023).
3 Leys, Tony. (2023). *Wave of Rural Nursing Home Closures Grows Amid Staff Crunch.* Kaiser Family Foundation. https://khn.org/news/article/ wave-of-rural-nursing-home-closures-grows-amid-staffing-crunch/. (accessed March 28, 2023).
4 Saric, Ivana. (2022). Nursing homes face closure risks amid staff shortages post-COVID. *Axios.* www.axios.com/2022/06/07/nursing-home-staff-shortage-closure-covid. (accessed March 28, 2023).
5 Hanna, Kerry, et al. (2022). Working in a care home during the COVID-19 pandemic: How has the pandemic changed working practices? A qualitive study. *BMC Geriatrics.* 22(129). https://doi.org/10.1186/ s12877-022-028222-0. (accessed January 2, 2023).
6 Taylor, Mariah. (2023). 128 nursing homes closed in 2022: Numbers by state. *Becker's Hospital Review.* www.beckershospitalreview.com/ post-acute/128-nursing-homes-closed-in-2022-numbers-by-states.html. (accessed April 3, 2023).
7 Carlton, Genevieve, PhD. (2023). Addressing the nursing home crisis: A new federal proposal makes nurses part of the solution. https:// nursejournal.org/articles/addressing-nursing-home-crisis/. (accessed October 17, 2023).
8 Kelleher, Olivia. (2022). Nursing home sector in 'crisis' as 17 facilities close in 2022 alone. *The Irish Times.* www.breakingnews.ie/ireland/nursing-home-sector-in-crisis-as-17facilities-close-in-2022-alone-1400972.html. (accessed March 29, 2023).
9 Parodi, Emilio. (2020). After coronavirus, Italian nursing homes face fight to survive. *Reuters.* www.reuters.com/article/ us-health-coronavirus-italy-nursinghomes-idUSKBN2320KG. (accessed March 29, 2023).
10 Spanko, Alex. (2020). HHS releases $4.9B in COVID-19 relief for skilled nursing facilities. https://skillednursingnews.com/2020/ 05/hhs-releases-4-9b-in-covid-19-relief-for-skilled-nursing-facilities/. (accessed November 1, 2023).
11 Goldstein, Matthew, et al. (2020). Pandemic's costs stagger the nursing home industry. *The New York Times.* https://www.nytimes. com/2020/04/21/business/coronavirus-nursing-home-finances.html. (accessed April 3, 2023).
12 American Healthcare Association. (2021). Transforming long term care: Maintaining minimum supply of personal protective equipment.

https://www.ahcancal.org/News-and-Communications/Press-Releases/Pages/Transforming-Long-Term-Care-Maintaining-Minimum-Supply-Of-Personal-Protective-equipment.aspx. (accessed April 3, 2023).

13 FEMA. (2020). PPE packages for nursing homes. www.fema.gov/fact-sheet/ppe-packages-nursing-homes. (accessed November 1, 2023).

14 Porter, Kristie, et al. (2022). *COVID-19 Pandemic Increased Nursing Homes' Reliance on Contract Staff to Address Staffing Shortages in 2020.* Department of Health and Human Services, Office of the Assistant Secretary for Planning and Evaluation. https://aspe.hhs.gov/sites/default/files/documents/f7c0751d7b3ae7337a3b5d5e3dcc2ae7/nh-reliance-contract-staff-brief.pdf. (accessed November 1, 2023). p. 2.

15 Stulick, Amy. (2021). Nursing homes use of staffing agencies soars during pandemic as workforce crisis deepens. *Skilled Nursing News*. https://skillednursingnews.com/2021/06/Nursing-homes-use-of-staffing-agencies-soars-during-pandemic-as-workforce-crisis-deepens/. (accessed April 3, 2023).

16 Musumeci, MaryBeth, et al. (2022). *State Actions to Address Nursing Home Staffing During COVID-19.* Kaiser Family Foundation. www.kff.org/medicaid/issue-brief/state-actions-to-address-nursing-home-staffing-during-covid-19/. (accessed April 3, 2023).

17 American Health Care Association. (2021). Nursing homes face imminent closures without financial support from congress. www.ahcancal.org/News-and-Communications/Press-Releases/Pages/Nursing-Homes-Face-Imminent-Closures-Without-Financial-Support-From-Congress.aspx. (accessed April 7, 2023).

18 Leys, Tony. (2023). *Wave of Rural Nursing Home Closures Grows Amid Staff Crunch.* Kaiser Family Foundation. https://khn.org/news/article/wave-of-rural-nursing-home-closures-grows-amid-staffing-crunch/. (accessed March 28, 2023).

19 American Healthcare Association. (2023). State of the nursing home Industry: Survey of 524 nursing home providers highlights persistent staffing and economic crisis. www.ahcancal.org/News-and-Communications/Fact-Sheets/FactSheets/SNF-Survey-December-2022.pdf. (accessed November 1, 2023).

20 Musumeci, MaryBeth, et al. (2022). *State Actions to Address Nursing Home Staffing During COVID-19.* Kaiser Family Foundation. www.kff.org/medicaid/issue-brief/state-actions-to-address-nursing-home-staffing-during-covid-19/. (accessed April 3, 2023).

21 Scales, Kezia, PhD. (2022). Essential support: State hazard pay and sick leave policies for direct care workers during COVD-19. www.phinational.org/resource/essential-support-state-hazard-pay-and-sick-leave-policies-for-direct-care-workers-during-covid-19/. (accessed November 1, 2023).

22 Kirzinger, Ashley, et al. (2021). *KFF/The Washington Post Frontline Health Care Workers Survey.* Kaiser Family Foundation. www.kff.org/coronavirus-covid-19/poll-finding/kff-washington-post-health-care-workers/. (accessed April 15, 2023).

23 Carlton, Genevieve, PhD. (2023). Addressing the nursing home crisis: A new federal proposal makes nurses part of the solution. https://nursejournal.org/articles/addressing-nursing-home-crisis/. (accessed October 17, 2023).

24 Department of Health. (2020). Minister for Health announces extension to the COVID-19 temporary assistance payment scheme. www.gov.ie/en/press-release/a3d4a-minister-for-health-announces-extension-to-the-covid-19-temporary-assistance-payment-scheme/#:~:text=As%20part%20of%20package%20of%20support%20measures%20for,which%20opened%20for%20applications%20on%2017%20April%202020. (accessed April 14, 2023).

25 HM Government. (2020). Care home support package. www.local.gov.uk/sites/default/files/documents/14%20May%202020%20-%20COVID-19%20Care%20home%20support%20package_0.pdf/. (accessed April 14, 2023).

26 Department of Health and Social Care. (2022). Increased funding for nursing in care homes. www.gov.uk/government/news/increased-funding-for-nursing-in-care-homes. (accessed April 14, 2023).

27 Department of Finance Canada. (2021). Fighting COVID-19. www.budgetcanada.ca/fes-eea/2020/report= rapport/chap1-en-html. (accessed April 14, 2023).

28 Seymour, Ron. (2020). Keeping health care workers static costs $10 million a month. *The Daily Courier*. www.kelowndailycourier.ca/news/article_cd62b3a4-7b4c-11wa-ad02-8fd2a425a6f9.html. (accessed April 14, 2023).

29 Grinspun, Doris, et al. (2023). COVID-19 pandemic in long-term care: An international perspective for policy consideration. *International Journal of Nursing Sciences*. www.ncbi.nlm.nih.gov/pmc/articles/PMC10063321/. (accessed April 14, 2023).

30 Williams, Gemma, et al. (2020). How are countries supporting their health workers during COVID-19? Data from the COVID-19 health system response monitor. *Eurohealth*. 26(2). www.ncbi.nlm.nih.gov/pmc/articles/PMC8574721/. (accessed April 24, 2023). p. 59.

31 Australian Government. (2021). My aged care. www.myagedcare.gov.au/aged-care-homes. (accessed April 1, 2023).

32 Australian Government, Department of Health. (2022). COVID-19 aged care support program extension.https://www.health.gov.au/news/announcements/extension-of-the-covid-19-aged-care-support-program-extension-grant-go4863. (accessed April 20, 2023).

33 Colombo, Francesca, et al. (2021). *Rising From the COVID-19 Crisis: Policy Responses in the Long-Term Care Sector*. Organisation for Economic Co-operation and Development (OECD). https://read.oecd-ilibrary.org/view/? ref=1122_1122652 – oyri4k81cp&title=Rising-from-the-COVID-19-crisis-policy-responses-in-the-long-term-care-sector. (accessed April 25, 2023). pp. 6, 7.

34 Colombo, Francesca, et al. (2021). *Rising From the COVID-19 Crisis: Policy Responses in the Long-Term Care Sector*. Organisation for Economic Co-operation and Development (OECD). https://read.

oecd-ilibrary.org/view/?ref=1122_1122652-oyri4k81cp&title=Rising-from-the-COVID-19-crisis-policy-responses-in-the-long-term-care-sector. (accessed April 25, 2023), pp. 6, 7.

35   Colombo, Francesca, et al. (2021). *Rising From the COVID-19 Crisis: Policy Responses in the Long-Term Care Sector.* Organisation for Economic Co-operation and Development (OECD). https://read. oecd-ilibrary.org/view/?ref=1122_1122652-oyri4k81cp&title=Rising-from-the-COVID-19-crisis-policy-responses-in-the-long-term-care-sector. (accessed April 25, 2023), pp. 6, 7.

36   Department of Health and Social Care. (2020). COVID-19: Our action plan for adult social care. www.gov.uk/government/publications/coronavirus-covid-19-adult-social-care-action-plan/covid-19-our-action-plan-for-adult-social-care. (accessed April 14, 2023).

37   Department of Health and Aged Care. (2023). Government support for providers and workers. www.health.gov.au/topics/aged-care/advice-on-aged-care-during-covid-19/government-supports.   (accessed April 18, 2023).

38   Colombo, Francesca, et al. (2021). *Rising From the COVID-19 Crisis: Policy Responses in the Long-Term Care Sector.* Organisation for Economic Co-operation and Development (OECD). https://read. oecd-ilibrary.org/view/?ref=1122_1122652-oyri4k81cp&title=Rising-from-the-COVID-19-crisis-policy-responses-in-the-long-term-care-sector. (accessed April 25, 2023). p. 8.

39   Colombo, Francesca, et al. (2021). *Rising From the COVID-19 Crisis: Policy Responses in the Long-Term Care Sector.* Organisation for Economic Co-operation and Development (OECD). https://read. oecd-ilibrary.org/view/?ref=1122_1122652-oyri4k81cp&title=Rising-from-the-COVID-19-crisis-policy-responses-in-the-long-term-care-sector. (accessed April 25, 2023). p. 8.

40   Department of Health and Aged Care. (2023). Government support for providers and workers. www.health. gov.au/topics/aged-care/advice-on-aged-care-during-covid-19/government-supports. (accessed April 18, 2023).

41   Colombo, Francesca, et al. (2021). *Rising From the COVID-19 Crisis: Policy Responses in the Long-Term Care Sector.* Organisation for Economic Co-operation and Development (OECD). https://read.oecd-ilibrary.org/view/?ref=1122_1122652-oyri4k81cp&title=Rising-from-the-COVID-19-crisis-policy-responses-in-the-long-term-care-sector. (accessed April 25, 2023), pp. 8–9.

42   Colombo, Francesca, et al. (2021). *Rising From the COVID-19 Crisis: Policy Responses in the Long-Term Care Sector.* Organisation for Economic Co-operation and Development (OECD). https://read.oecd-ilibrary.org/view/? ref=1122_1122652-oyri4k81cp&title=Rising-from-the-COVID-19-crisis-policy-responses-in-the-long-term-care-sector. (accessed April 25, 2023). p. 9.

43   Flynn, Maggie. (2021). Staffing and ownership structure take center stage in senate hearing on COVID-19 in nursing homes. *Skilled Nursing News.* https://skillednursingnews.com/2021/03/staffing-and-ownership-structure-

take-center-stage-in-senate-hearing-on-covid-19-in-nursing-homes/. (accessed April 7, 2023).

44 Taylor, Kristin. (2020). Statutory protection from COVID-19 related liability. https://cassels.com/insights/statutory-protection-from-covid-19-related-liability/. (accessed May 2, 2023).

45 The Network for Public Health Law. (2023). Garcia v. Welltower OpCo Group, LLC et al. www.networkforphl.org/resources/garcia-v-welltower-opco-group-llc-et-al/. (accessed May 6, 2023).

46 Pierson, Brenda. (2022). U.S. Supreme Court rebuffs dispute over nursing home COVID suits. *Reuters News*. https://www.reuters.com/legal/us-supreme-court-rebuffs-dispute-over-nursing-home-covid-suits-2022-11-21/. (accessed May 6, 2023).

47 Lependorf and Silverstein. (2022). More nursing homes in New Jersey raise serious questions. www.lependorf.com/blog/wrongful-death/nursing-home-lawsuits-new-jersey-raise-questions/. (accessed May 6, 2023).

48 Difilippo, Dana. (2022). New lawsuits over New Jersey nursing home COVID-19 deaths claim 'state-created danger'. *Philly Voice*. www.phillyvoice.com/new-jersey-covid-19-nursing-home-lawsuit-phil-murphy-judith-persichilli/. (accessed May 6, 2023).

49 Shaw, Adam. (2023). Ex-Gov. Andrew Cuomo faces new lawsuit alleging 'unmitigated greed' contributed to nursing home death. *Fox News*. https://flipboard.com/@foxnews/politics-i8p0v8l2z/-/a-Rnpc4X7uSQuwV01 ioiR0dQ%3Aa%3A47769551-%2F0#:~:text= Former%20 New%20 York%20Gov.%20Andrew%20Cuomo%20is%20facing,and%20" un-mitigated%20greed"%20had%20led%20to%20needless%20deaths. (accessed May 6, 2023).

50 Rubinkam, Michael. (2020). Pennsylvania nursing home sued over severe COVID-19 outbreak. *WTAE*. https://www.wtae.com/article/brighton-rehab-lawsuit-alleges-nursing-home-responsible-covid-19-deaths/34431214. (accessed May 6, 2023).

51 Chen, Stacy. (2020). Family files 1st wrongful death lawsuit against Life Care Center in Washington over coronavirus outbreak. *ABC News*. https://abcnews.go.com/Health/family-files-1st-wrongful-death-lawsuit-life-care/story?id=70122496. (accessed May 6, 2023).

52 Department of Justice. (2022). MorseLife nursing home health system agrees to pay 1.75 million to settle false claims act allegations for facilitating COVID-19 vaccinations of ineligible donors and prospective donors. www.justice.gov/opa/pr/morselife-nursing-home-health-system-agrees-pay-175-million-settle-false-claims-act. (accessed May 6, 2023).

53 Blackwell, Tom. (2023). 'Gross negligence': Judge gives go-ahead to COVID-deaths Lawsuit against Ontario. *National Post*. https://national-post.com/news/covid-deaths-lawsuit-against-ontario. (accessed May 6, 2023).

54 Carswell, Simon. (2022). Co Louth nursing home being sued over COVID-19 death. *The Irish Times*. https://www.irishtimes.com/news/health/co-louth-nursing-home-being-sued-over-covid-19-death-1.4836487.(accessed May 6, 2023).

55 Horgan-Jones, Jack. (2022). Wrongful death claim made against nursing home hit by COVID. *The Irish Times*. https://www.irishtimes.
   com/news/health/wrongful-death-claim-made-against-nursing-
   home-hit-by-covid-19-1.4813680. (accessed May 6, 2023).
56 Feely, Kieran. (2022). Nursing home deaths and the search for accountability. *Medical Independent*. www.medicalindependent.ie/in-the-news/
   news-features/nursing-home-deaths-and-the-search-for-accountability/.
   (accessed May 6, 2023).
57 Reuters. (2020). Spain's Supreme Court orders probe into nursing home
   COVID-19 deaths. www.reuters.com/business/healthcare-pharmaceuticals/
   spains-supreme-court-orders-probe-into-nursing-home-covid-19-
   deaths-2020-12-18/. (accessed May 6, 2023).

Section II

Structural, Policy, and Procedural Changes for Improvement of Surveillance, Mitigation, and Quality of Care

3 LTC Improved Infection Surveillance, Control, and Prevention Strategies

When the March 13, 2020, memorandum on COVID from the CMS was issued, each state's HHS entity that inspects nursing homes began a process of notification through protocols, policies, and procedures to all facilities in their region. CMS provided multiple *COVID-19 Long-Term Care Facility Guidance* protocols, many times in conjunction with the CDC. These protocols, practices, and procedures are utilized for all pandemics and consist of similar mitigation strategies in many countries; thus, they need to be evaluated and discussed to improve IPC mitigation strategies in nursing homes for future public health emergencies.

Phase I: Initial Mitigation Strategies

The phase I mitigation strategy for LTC in the United States was to deter the initial transmission of COVID-19 into the facilities. As we all know, this objective was not obtained, even with the implementation of strict restrictive facility entrance protocols.

As previously stated, the majority of outbreaks in care facilities were initiated by asymptomatic employees, even with mask mandates. The CDC does agree that wearing a mask decreases the odds of getting COVID, yet it does not completely eradicate the potential. Surgical masks decrease the odds of testing positive for COVID by 66% and N95 masks lowered the odds by 88%.[1]

Restrictions

In the United States, during the early phase of the pandemic, nursing homes sent out letters of notification to all family members about visitor restrictions and education about the SARS-CoV-2 virus. All residents were notified of visitor restrictions via verbal communication, education was provided with regard to the COVID-19 virus, and alternate forms of communication such as face-time, zoom, phone calls, letters, and text messaging were discussed with patients.

DOI: 10.4324/9781003466192-6

Social Services was highly involved in assisting residents to sustain familial contact through alternate channels, attempting to ensure the maintenance of psychological and emotional health. Some organizations donated ipads to nursing homes for clients, so they could have their own e-source for familial contact purposes. Isolation (visitor restriction) signs were posted throughout each facility and main entrance doors were constantly locked to deter people from entering facilities unnoticed.

All nonessential personnel were restricted from entering nursing homes nationwide, which in many cases entailed physicians, pharmacists, dieticians, psychologists, surveyors, corporate executives, clergy, regional nurses, and so on. Zoom, telehealth, and telemental health became highly utilized alternative sources to meet residents' healthcare requirements during the pandemic. Narcotic medication destruction with the pharmacist was conducted via video conferences and was videotaped for substantiating evidence of the procedure. Annual nursing home inspections were placed on hold during the initial phase of the pandemic, and early pandemic restrictions limited the surveyors' contact with nursing homes.

Communal activities such as group dining, group activities, religious services, and so on were eradicated, and each client was encouraged to remain in their room. Activity Directors had to incorporate other alternatives to meet each client's psychosocial needs—music was utilized in many facilities—via intercoms, karaoke machines, and CD players. Hall bingo with social distancing occurred in some nursing homes. And, the activities department also provided 1:1 conversations (with social distancing) for residents in many instances.

Almost all countries initiated strict IPC restrictions for nursing homes in March 2020. Australia's initial government mitigation strategies for nursing homes included both funding and policy measures and limited visitation in care homes restricting the visit episodes to private rooms only and limiting the number to two individuals per day. The Dutch government, Japan, and Turkey's Ministry of Family, Labour, and Social Services implemented strict prevention and protection measures in care facilities including suspended visitation. Italy implemented their mitigation intervention for LTC suspending visitation and pre-established operational guidelines for nursing homes were updated and released by the Ministry of Health.

And, in Chile, the COVID-19 response began with the Ministry of Health, the National Service for Older People, and the Chilean Geriatrics and Gerontology Society working together to coordinate the implementation of IPC measures in LTC. All LTC facilities banned visitation and halted admissions.

Restriction Protocols for Future Pandemics

As discussed in Chapter 1, the strict isolative procedures elicited many physical and psychological burdens for the gerontological client. It is perceived by many healthcare professionals that the length of time residents were mandated to maintain the isolation, adversely impacted their health. Potentially, for future pandemics, the process of providing enhanced PPE to residents could be implemented to deter transmission, thus allowing them to come out of their rooms within a shorter time span, promoting mental and physical well-being.

Also, the restriction of nonessential employees for a long period of time impacted care provisions in some facilities; state surveyors, dieticians, pharmacists, and mental health providers not regularly providing consultation contributed to some adversities. In addition, clergy being restricted from nursing homes impacted the spiritual well-being of some residents. For future pandemics, the time span for such strict restrictions with regard to facility accessibility for the perceived nonessential employees should be evaluated, since most facilities did provide rigorous screening upon entrance to a facility. Restrictions, screening, and isolation units were included in the mitigation plan, all LTC facilities in the United States had to develop a facility-specific mitigation plan.

Mitigation Plan

A *mitigation plan* is a formulation of steps and/or processes that assist in decreasing the potential of risk/harm or the impact of risk/harm from specific sources, such as a pandemic. A typical mitigation plan for SARS-CoV-2 in nursing homes defined processes to implement and monitor in the areas of cleaning/disinfection, PPE, screening, visitation, testing, isolation, cohorting, reporting, surveillance, workforce and staffing, infection control teams, communication, transportation, and education/training. The mitigation plans were submitted to each state's Department of HHS and after approval from the state were implemented to decrease the risk or impact of COVID-19 in nursing homes.

Educational Needs for Future Pandemic Mitigation Plans

For future pandemics, there should be mandatory educational processes with regard to the mitigation plan for all employees in nursing homes. Most facilities provided a copy to staff for reference, but no formal education on the plan was provided in a lot of elder care homes. Providing formal documented education on mitigation strategies to decrease the potential of transmission, including education on specific restrictions and screening, could potentially lower the risk and impact of infection processes during a pandemic.

Screening Processes

Initial screening processes were implemented for all employees and other individuals entering a facility (i.e., ambulance personnel, mortician) in the United States. Screening consisted of checking the temperature and having the person answer questions with regard to COVID signs and symptoms and potential for exposure—such as traveling to another country or having contact with a COVID-positive individual.

There was some variance between states in America on how this process was conducted, many nursing homes just screened individuals upon entering the facility, but some also conducted a screening process when individuals left the building. The sources for the screening processes varied too; some facilities utilized a hard copy paper written process, while others utilized electronic methods to record the data. There was also variance in the actual screening conduction, some facilities allowed self-screening, while others implemented specific staff members to perform the screening protocols. In any of the processes, if an individual had been exposed to COVID or had signs and symptoms of COVID, they were not allowed to enter the facility.

Initial screening protocols for patients were established also, at first, it was a temperature and assessing for signs and symptoms of SARS-CoV-2 every 24 hours. Most facilities initiated with a hard copy assessment process but quickly developed a system in Point-Click-Care (e-medical record documentation) to conform with CMS guidelines. As positive cases developed in facilities, the screening of clients increased up to the implementation of every four-hour screening protocol for patients who had been exposed to a positive COVID-19 individual. Turkey's Ministry of Family, Labour, and Social Services and Chile also initiated monitoring of residents (symptom checks) and suspected cases were transferred to the hospital.

Screening Procedures for Future Pandemics

Due to staffing problems, there was a lot of controversy in most LTC facilities as to how to conduct the screening processes. Again, some facilities implemented an electronic screening device that allowed for self-screening for both employees and others entering the facility that has been perceived by many to be the most effective procedural system for this process. To prepare for future pandemics, the industry should ensure that each facility has an electronic screening device on hand and that PRN (as needed) certified nursing assistants and licensed nurses are available to assist with the daily screening of residents.

Isolation Units

Red COVID Isolation Units were established in all nursing homes throughout the United States. These units were sectioned off and designated for positive SARS-CoV-2 clients on contact and droplet precautions. Each red isolation unit was supposed to have its own separate entrance and exit from the facility,

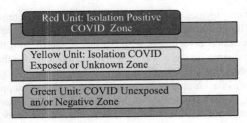

Figure 3.1 COVID Isolation Zones.

without having contact with other areas of the facility. As stated in the introduction, in some facilities, the architecture of the buildings made it hard, if not impossible, to establish an area of this nature. Figure 3.1 illustrates the isolation zones in LTC facilities.

As time progressed, nursing homes were also separated into Green and Yellow Units. Green Units contained clients who were COVID-negative and had not been exposed (or potentially exposed) to the virus and Yellow Units contained clients who were COVID-negative but were within 14 days of exposure (or potential exposure).

All new admissions went to the Yellow Units (for 14 days) as they were in the community or the hospital and exposure to asymptomatic individuals was unknown. Again, this process did pose a few difficulties in some facilities because of the architectural design of the facilities.

Implementation of Infection Control Zones for Future Pandemics

With regard to future protocols established on this procedure, all infection preventionists (IPs) need to be well-educated on how to designate the separation of red, yellow, and green units and need to provide that education to staff, so the entire facility can assist with decreasing risk for transmission. By effectively separating areas of the nursing home based on the level of perceived exposure or potential exposure; transmissions could potentially be more controlled, and the process could also assist in enforcing the utilization of appropriate PPE for each zone.

Personal Protective Equipment

Mandatory PPE was implemented; initially, it was a surgical mask and increased hand hygiene for both patients and employees in US facilities. As positive cases developed in LTC environments: gowns, gloves, face shields, goggles, and N95 masks were incorporated into daily utilization. The addition of face shield employment in nursing homes assisted in decreasing percentages for COVID transmission even more. One study identified a reduction of COVID transmission percentages with the utilization of both the mask and face shield concurrently; there was a 98% reduction level for the face shield and a 97.3% reduction level for the mask.[2]

A person was designated in each facility to track PPE supply and utilization. Again, in the early stages of the pandemic, there was a shortage of N95 masks and hand sanitizers which led to some controversy in America. Some corporations were utilizing the process of borrowing from sister facilities to meet the demand of supplies until alternate supply sources could be located.

Italy experienced an extreme shortage of PPE and nursing homes were not given priority for supplies. It is the responsibility of each regional health entity (Aziende Sanitaire Locali, Italian Ministry of Health) to assist their LTC sector; most enacted late without any clear instructions from the national level.[3] And, the Dutch government identified the lack of PPE availability as one major factor in deterring transmission within the industry in this country and it has been identified by the government that the supply of PPE to LTC is as important as acute care.[4]

Ensure PPE Stock Pile and Availability for Future Pandemics

The worldwide reports of PPE shortages resulted in many HCWs being placed at increased risk due to inadequate PPE availability. The key to any pandemic preparedness plan is to be proactive. A prevention investment that is widely recognized to be crucial is the stockpiling of PPE for essential workers. The primary purpose of a stockpile is to ensure sufficient PPE to protect the health of essential workers.

The quantity of PPE stockpiled depends on predictions of a "burn rate" of PPE use during a pandemic. Because a stockpile is a form of insurance protection during low probability, but potential emergencies, a stockpile that ensures generous availability of PPE at burn rates similar to the early period of COVID-19 is essential.

Waiting to place orders just before or even during a pandemic is not a smart strategy, the ideal time to plan and place pandemic stockpile orders is during the spring and summer months. To best determine the quantity that a facility would need, the CDC recommends stockpiling enough supplies for the duration of a pandemic wave, which is estimated to last between six and eight weeks.

A California Health Care Foundation survey conducted from June 5 to July 12, 2020, among California skilled nursing facility staff found that more than 90 days into the COVID-19 pandemic, more than 20% of respondents still reported inadequate PPE, and more than 80% were very or extremely concerned about workplace infection. California Senate Bill 275 as amended in July 2020 requires the state to create a PPE stockpile sufficient to protect healthcare and other essential workers for at least 90 days for any future pandemic or health emergency.[5]

Most of the PPE used in Europe is produced offshore, and there is a high reliance on a few global suppliers. Medical face masks, which are almost exclusively produced in China, were in short supply during the COVID-19 pandemic in many industrialized countries, which do not produce them. Strict lockdowns and other pandemic-related restrictions imposed in supplier countries exacerbated the situation.[6]

The shortages drove many domestic companies to rapidly reconfigure their supply chains. For example, an article in 2021 reported that the manufacturing of facemasks in China rose from 20 million facemasks per day on January 14 to about 116 million per day at the end of February.[7] In the United Kingdom, there were several organizations that repurposed their existing manufacturing facilities to make PPE.[8] For example, the British fashion retailer Barbour started producing protective gowns. Burberry retooled its trench coat factory to non-surgical gowns and masks for patients.[9] Louis Vuitton also started producing masks for frontline workers and Dior switched to the production of hydro-alcoholic gel hand sanitizers.[10] Such innovations enabled firms to extend their supply chains by creating separate channels of supply through the use of alternative and in some cases local providers or by restructuring international purchasing operations.

A Scottish survey on perceptions with regard to ensuring PPE stockpiles was conducted and revealed that many individuals in Scotland felt that a Scottish stockpile would help ensure that Scotland has adequate access to PPE based on its own needs as distinct from the rest of the United Kingdom, the following are a few of the responses in the survey:

> It makes sense for Scotland to have its own stockpile that is more easily accessible to Scottish organizations and which is planned appropriately for a Scottish context, for instance mindful of the make-up of the social care sector in Scotland.
>
> —Scottish Care[11]

> A Scottish stockpile of PPE would offer the advantages of PPE being held at a more 'local' level which would potentially speed up response times if needed.
>
> —Aberdeenshire HSCP[12]

> Local stockpiling and management of PPE supplies would avoid a repeat of the distribution issues which hindered the delivery of health and social care services during the Covid-19 pandemic.
>
> —Leonard Cheshire in Scotland[13]

Also, a few respondents felt that a Scottish approach could be more cost-effective than, or mitigate against, international supply chains that can be volatile and unreliable. In the United States, it is mandatory for every nursing home facility to retain a full-time IP on staff as this person assists with PPE utilization compliance.

Infection Preventionist

In LTC, the IP is a nurse who has received additional training (certification) in the branch of IPC and ensures staff are following protocols to deter infection transmission. The CDC offers a 23-module course online specifically for nursing home IP positions that cover core activities of an effective IPC program including, recommended practices to decrease pathogen transmission, health-care-associated infections, and antibiotic resistance. During the pandemic, the IP was a core source for ongoing strategies to deter the transmission of COVID-19 in facilities.

Improved IPC Education

Ongoing, infection control education is a necessity in all healthcare settings. When infection prevention practitioners are educating and influencing HCWs, compliance with the IPC guidance provided is a necessity, and educative efforts must be repeated and performed as part of a collaborative and multidimensional approach. In the United States, the IP in each facility is responsible for the ongoing educational processes and systems to monitor for compliance.

The CDC offers a tool to assess compliance called the Infection Control Assessment and Response (ICAR) Tool for General IPC Across Settings. ICAR tools are used to systematically assess a healthcare facility's IPC practices and guide quality improvement activities (e.g., by addressing identified gaps).

Nursing homes may decide whether to use the tool in its entirety or select among the pool of questions that best fit their jurisdictional needs and priorities as part of quality improvement efforts. The decision to conduct an assessment in-person or remotely via a Tele-ICAR depends upon several factors, such as available public health resources, the location and remoteness of the facility, and the presence of an active outbreak. For facilities with recent cases of SARS-CoV-2 infection in healthcare personnel or residents, an in-person assessment is preferred; however, jurisdictions must individually determine how to best provide assistance in the timeliest manner.[14]

AUSTRALIA

The Australian Clinical Excellence Commission provided an updated document that contains recommendations relating to IPC measures for COVID-19 and other acute respiratory infections (ARIs) in healthcare settings. Residential aged care facilities (RACF), and community residential care group homes are congregate settings that are included with specific emphasis on COVID-19 and influenza. Principles can be applied as required to respiratory syncytial virus (RSV) and other respiratory pathogens. The manual aligns with the principles outlined in the New South Wales Infection Prevention and Control Policy Directive and is consistent with the principles and practices within the Infection Prevention and Control Practice Handbook. The guidance in this Manual also includes IPC best practice information on COVID-19 and other ARIs, based on the known transmission characteristics, and is also responsive to the changing incidence and burden of infection in the health system.[15]

CANADA

In Canada, Public Health Ontario issued "Infection Prevention and Control for Long-Term Care Homes" in December 2020. The Department of Health and Wellness in Nova Scotia released *Guidelines for Long-Term Care Facilities* for Nova Scotia in December 2020. In New Brunswick, the Department of Social Development provided directives in July 2022 through *Living with COVID: management of COVID-19 for New Brunswick Long Term Care Homes* and *COVID-19 Guidance for Long-Term Care Facilities (LTCF)*, which was released in April 2020 from the Office of the Chief Medical Officer of Health. The Ministry of Long-Term Care issued guidance in January 2021, *IPC program guidance* for regular operations and outbreak conditions in Canadian care homes.

UNITED KINGDOM

The NHS England updated their IPC guidance in 2023, via the *National infection prevention and control manual for England*. The manual contains evidence-based practices for use by all those involved in care provision in England and should be adopted as guidance in NHS settings or settings where NHS services are delivered and the principles should be applied in all care settings to ensure a consistent UK-wide approach to IPC; however, some operational and organizational details may differ across the nations.

The UK utilizes IPC teams that are directed to engage with staff to develop systems and processes that lead to sustainable and reliable improvements in applying IPC practices. The qualified IPC staff provide expert advice on applying IPC in nursing homes and on individual risk assessments, ensuring that action is taken as required. In addition, the IP teams maintain that nursing home staff providing care show their understanding by applying IPC principles in the work environment and maintain competence, skills, and knowledge in IPC by attending educational events and/or completing training.[16]

SPAIN

The Spanish Minister of Health released guidance for LTC facilities in March 2020, *Prevention and control guidelines against COVID-19 in nursing homes and other residential social services centers.*

Public and State Health Departments

Local and state health departments became a common resource for the IP in nursing homes in the United States. These entities also provided direction on emergency preparedness and response, assessment and surveillance, and communications. In one nursing home, the IP was trained by the public health department on how to perform COVID testing. The local health department also came to the nursing home to give recommendations with regard to the development of specified units/zones and provided some of the needed supplies for client and staff testing.

Public health was a common resource for questions with regard to admissions, readmissions, longevity of isolation, client transfers, and in some cases attempting to locate additional staff to work in nursing homes. Even being short-staffed and many times out-resourced themselves, the public health departments did everything they could to assist the LTC industry in mitigating SARS-CoV-2 in the United States.

Phase II: Intermediate Mitigation Strategies

America continued with additional strategies to deter transmission of SARS-CoV-2 in elder care facilities with the addition of protocols for SARS-CoV-2 surveillance testing of both staff and residents. There were initially two types of testing; nucleic acid amplification tests (polymerase chain reaction (PCR) tests) and antigen tests (rapid). The rapid test detects protein fragments specific to the coronavirus, while the PCR test detects ribonucleic acid (RNA) that is specific to the COVID virus.

At first, the PCR testing was conducted by outside entities for staff and patients, such as public health departments. Again, public health departments in the initial stages also assisted with procuring the needed supplies for sample collection and training staff on how to perform COVID testing via the nasal swab procedure. After appropriate training and obtaining the Clinical Laboratory Improvements Amendments (CLIA law), Certificate of Waiver, HCWs in LTC would perform the nasal swab procedure for both clients and employees and transport the specimens to the public health department lab for evaluation. Initially, all individuals in an LTC facility were SARS-CoV-2 tested one time per week. At this point, there was approximately a two- to three-day turn-around period for obtaining test results.

Point-of-care testing was eventually introduced into LTC facilities with the US Department of HHS initially distributing the Quidel Sofia 2 or BD Veritor

Plus instruments and supplies to utilize in nursing homes for SARS-CoV-2 surveillance testing purposes. The rapid antigen point-of-care testing kits named Celtrion Dia and Abbot BinaxNOW were utilized most frequently after being available on the market mostly related to cost factors. The implementation of these testing instruments decreased test result turn-around time to 15–20 minutes. As more positive cases developed, the SARS-CoV-2 testing increased to two times per week for both employees and residents.

COVID Surveillance in Other Countries

Surveillance testing for SARS-CoV-2 and reporting of cases varied in other countries. Higher-income countries incorporated more mitigation processes than middle- and low-income countries. Also, in many countries, acute care was given priority over LTC in terms of supplies and clearly defined policies and procedures for IPC.

Canada

In November 2020, the Canadian Minister of Health established the COVID-19 Testing and Screening Expert Advisory Panel. The panel members' initial recommendations for LTC were to test frequently utilizing rapid tests for screening and to confirm positive cases with PCR testing as appropriate. Each province in Canada established their testing protocols; in Ontario, rapid antigen testing was made mandatory by mid-March 2021 for any individual who entered a nursing facility, including volunteers and family members. Full-time staff were required to be tested three times per week and other individuals anytime they entered the nursing home.[17]

United Kingdom

The English Government initiated COVID test kit deliveries in April 2020, to specific care homes under a satellite program. Then in May 2020, the Department of Health and Social Care for the United Kingdom announced a new online portal for nursing homes to obtain point-of-care rapid testing supplies for testing of symptomatic and non-symptomatic residents and staff. Prior to May 2020, those individuals not in the satellite program were tested by Public Health England or drive-thru-testing sites when an outbreak occurred in a nursing home.

Spain

COVID-19 tests were not commonly or consistently conducted at nursing homes in Spain in April 2020, primarily because of a nationwide shortage of testing kits. Spain's Minister of Health, Salvador Illa, announced on April 5 that a million rapid diagnostic tests would be distributed among autonomous communities to tackle the problem. The Spanish authorities recommended carrying out diagnostic tests, prioritizing health and socio-health, arranging educational centers, as well as prioritizing vulnerable patients. Thus, in nursing homes, during an outbreak, it may be advised to obtain PCR tests from all residents and employees.[18]

The last recommendation in May 2022 from the Ministry of Health of Castilla Mancha (Spain) was that employees of health and socio-health centers are considered suspected cases of COVID-19 if they present compatible symptoms. In addition, they recommended performing two weekly SARS-CoV-2 Rapid Antigen Nasal Tests in unvaccinated employees (even if they do not have symptoms or have had no close contacts) and PCR testing three to five days after a positive close contact with COVID-19.[19]

Italy and Netherlands

In Italy, testing for COVID-19 was heavily rationed with supplies concentrated on acute care sectors. In the nursing home industry, only symptomatic residents and HCWs were provided COVID testing in the first part of April 2020, and RT-PCR testing was incorporated for employees only by the end of April.[20] Additionally, testing for COVID-19 was initiated in the Netherlands on April 6, 2020, for hospital staff and suspected cases—it later expanded to LTC workers demonstrating symptoms of COVID.[21]

Reporting

In the United States, reporting of all SARS-CoV-2 test results was incorporated at the state level and later to the NHSN (CDC). It was implemented as a weekly reporting process entailing positive and negative testing results, PPE utilization and supplies, staffing, hospitalizations, isolation precautions, deaths, ventilator capacity, the number of suspected positive cases, and resident beds/census. Most facilities reported to both entities (state and CDC), but California devised an online reporting system that was linked to the CDC for the state level to transfer the information, so only one data entry had to be inputted to provide the regulated information.

COVID reporting to residents, family members, and representatives was also incorporated into facility protocols in the United States. Any positive case or any situation of three individuals with new onset of respiratory signs and symptoms occurring within 72 hours of each other was relayed to customers by 5:00 P.M. the following day. Some facilities implemented an automatic reporting system to representatives and families through cell phones; this process was usually established and maintained by the administrator of a facility. However, many facilities made personal phone calls to provide the required information to representatives and family members. Residents who were deemed to have capacity were verbally informed of the required COVID information. Figure 3.2 illustrates positive COVID cases in US nursing homes.

In Canada, reporting of nursing home-positive COVID cases was conducted with each jurisdiction's public health authority. Again, the death rates of residents in LTC in Ontario, Canada, initiated the Fixing Long-Term Care Act 2021, S, O, 2021, c. 39, Sched, which increased fines and impeded the government from taking possession of a nursing home if regulations were not met. All COVID testing in LTC was reported to the UK Health Security Agency (UKHSA) weekly for negative results, and positive results needed to be reported within 24 hours.

Infection Control Inspections/Surveys

All previously implemented mitigation strategies were carried over to phase II. As stated earlier, all annual surveys were eradicated during the lockdown, but infection control surveys became a common occurrence in LTC during this time period. The title "COVID-19 Focused Survey" was given to the inspection process. New F tags were implemented for this infection control survey:

- F884-Reporting to CDC
- F885-Reporting to Residents, their Representatives, and Families

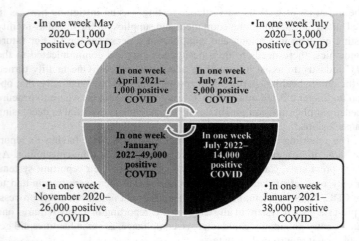

Figure 3.2 Positive Resident COVID Cases in US Nursing Homes.[22]

Source: Centers for Medicare & Medicaid Services. This is a rectangular art design with a center circle that shows the actual number of positive COVID cases in US nursing homes in one week, with the lowest number in April 2021 at 1,000 cases and the highest in one week in January 2022 at 49,000 cases.

The main objectives for the surveyors were to ensure that IPC strategies were effective through: the utilization of standard and transmission-based precautions, quality of resident care demonstrated acceptable practices, a surveillance plan was implemented and carried out, the facility was following visitation protocols, screening processes were conducted, education was provided, protocols for reporting were followed, and staffing policies and procedures addressed shortages.

By August 18, 2020, approximately 99.2% of American nursing homes had at least one infection control survey conducted. CMS reported that 180 "immediate jeopardy" deficiencies were cited, meaning noncompliance with regulations that had caused or was likely to cause serious injury/harm was substantiated. Civil monetary penalties were imposed for these deficiencies, encompassing approximately $10 million in fines. It was also identified that a few nursing homes were not compliant with reporting COVID data to the CDC and that process entailed $5.5 million in civil penalties.[23]

The CQC conducted IPC inspections of care homes during the COVID-19 pandemic. And in Italy, an organization called Nuclei Antisofisticazioni e Sanita (NAS) apparently is the healthcare police that investigated several nursing homes during the pandemic, due to complaints.

Improved Testing, Reporting, and IC Surveys for Future Pandemics

The initiation of COVID surveillance testing was an intriguing process in the United States. Obtaining equipment and supplies for the initial in-facility testing evolved into a long and complicated process for the IP. For future pandemics, there needs to be a designated supplier communicated to the LTC industry to assist in providing adequate services. One facility turned to the public health department for testing supplies, but eventually, that option no longer existed either. Effective communication on where to procure needed supplies and equipment during a pandemic is essential to decreasing transmissions.

The reporting process could be improved upon also; having to report the same information into two different databases is time-consuming. As stated previously, California did eventually develop their reporting system, so only one set of data entries was required that then were transmitted to the CDC, NHSN system, but some other states did not develop this process. A pre-established system in all states for IPC reporting that only requires one dataset entry potentially could improve compliance, as some facilities did get fined for not reporting their data.

Increased IPC surveys in nursing homes during a pandemic could impact compliance in facilities that are identified as problematic in the United States and throughout the world. By frequently visiting these facilities and imposing sanctions for non-compliance, there could potentially be a decrease in transmission rates and improvement with regard to mortality and morbidity in these facilities.

Phase III: Final Mitigation Strategies

The vaccination process to assist in obtaining SARS-CoV-2 herd immunity was initiated in LTC facilities in December 2020. In America, local pharmacies, such as CVS, administered the immunizations to residents and employees. However, nursing home healthcare professionals had to devise the list of patients and employees; obtain all the consents; provide the necessary educational protocols; assess for potential adversities to receive the vaccination related to diagnosis, medications, allergies, and so on; set up the medical areas for the vaccination clinic to be conducted; obtain the necessary vital signs prior to administration; and assist the pharmacists on the day of the immunization clinic. Figures 3.3 and 3.4 depict some of the American states' vaccination completion percentages for residents.

Many nursing homes had the Moderna mRNA COVID-19 vaccine administered. The Pfizer-BioNTech COVID-19 vaccine was also available on the market at the initiation of vaccination processes in nursing homes. According to CMS, in October 2022, the national percentage of residents with complete

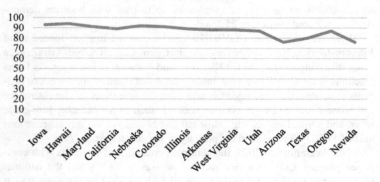

Percentage of Resident Primary COVID-19 Vaccination

Figure 3.3 October 2022, Percentage of Primary COVID-19 Vaccination Completed in US Nursing Homes.[24]

Source: Centers for Medicare & Medicaid Services. This is a line graph illustrating a vertical axis of percentages from 0% to 100% and a horizontal axis listing specific US states, showing the percentage of COVID primary vaccination series completed for residents by October 2022, with Iowa at the highest rate and Arizona at the lowest.

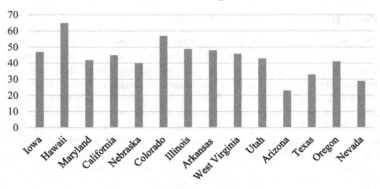

Percentage of Resident COVID-19 Boosters Completed

Figure 3.4 October 2022, Percentage of COVID-19 Boosters Completed in US Nursing Homes.[26]

Source: Centers for Medicare & Medicaid Services. This is a column graph with a vertical axis showing percentages from 0% to 70% and a horizontal axis listing specific US states, representing resident COVID booster vaccination, with Hawaii at the highest percentage and Arizona at the lowest.

primary vaccination was 86.9%, residents who were up-to-date with boosters had a national rate of 39.5%, employees with complete primary vaccination was at 86.7% nationally, and employees up to date with boosters demonstrated a national average at 25.2%.[25]

There are some other COVID-19 vaccines on the market: Johnson and Johnson-Janssen, Novavax-Nuvaxovid and Covovax, and Oxford-AstraZeneca being distributed in the United Kingdom and some other countries. As far as reactions to the COVID vaccine, most individuals whether employees or residents experienced a sore injection arm after the first vaccine administration, and some developed mild symptomatology such as a headache, low-grade fever, and generalized aching. Most nursing homes had no serious reactions to the COVID-19 vaccine in the primary or booster stages.

In the beginning of 2023, the national percentage of residents with completed primary COVID series vaccination was at 84.8% and the national percentage of residents up-to-date with all SARS-CoV-2 vaccinations was at 55.2% in the United States. Staff vaccination rates were at 85.8% for the primary COVID series and 23% for staff being up-to-date with their vaccinations as of April 30, 2023.[27]

In Figure 3.5, the resident percentage of primary vaccination rates is presented in specific states. In September 2023, CMS data revealed that 61.7% of

Resident Percentage of Primary COVID
Vaccination Completed, 2023

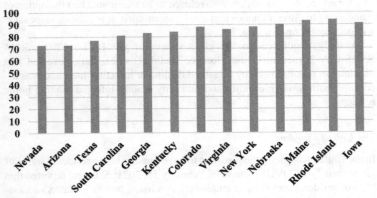

Figure 3.5 US Resident Primary Series COVID Vaccination Rates.[29]

Source: Centers for Disease Control and Prevention. This is a column graph illustrating a vertical axis of percentages from 0% to 100% and a horizontal axis listing specific US states, showing completed resident COVID primary vaccination by April 2023, with Nevada at the lowest percentage rate and Rhode Island at the highest.

nursing home residents were up-to-date with COVID vaccines, and 25.5% of staff in LTC were up-to-date with the vaccination series.[28]

Other Countries

Other countries, just like the United States, identified that the gerontological population in nursing homes and the staff that care for them should be given first priority for the COVID-19 vaccination. In March 2021, some Canadian Provinces reported high rates of primary vaccination initiation with 91–95% of residents in British Colombia, Quebec, Ontario, Saskatchewan, and Nova Scotia receiving their first COVID vaccine dose, while other Provinces did not report their nursing home data including Alberta, Manitoba, Newfoundland, Labrador, New Brunswick, Yukon, and Nunavut.[30]

Ontario, Canada, reported vaccination results in an article *Early Impact of Ontario's COVID-19 Vaccine Rollout on Long-Term Care Home Residents and Health Care Workers*, stating that as of February 23, 2021, COVID-19 vaccination in LTC homes prevented an estimated 2,079 SARS-CoV-2 infections, 249 COVID-19 hospitalizations, and 615 COVID-19 deaths regarding residents.[31]

Italy

Italy was the first European country to make COVID-19 vaccination mandatory for all HCWs, employees who refused to be vaccinated had the option of transferring to different duties that deter transmission or to choose suspension without pay for up to a year.[32]

A study conducted on the effectiveness of the BNT 162b2 mRNA SARS-CoV-2 vaccine in the Florence Health District, Italy, revealed that vaccination was followed by a marked decline in infection rates and was associated with lower morbidity and mortality among infected nursing home residents.[33]

The United Kingdom

In the United Kingdom, the goal was to have nursing home residents and staff given their first COVID vaccine by February 15, 2021; Scotland reported that 98% of residents and 88% of employees in nursing homes initiated vaccination, approximately 75% of residents in Wales elder care nursing facilities had their first dose, and Northern Ireland stated that 100% of their care homes initiated administration of the first dose.[34]

Australia

A dataset for Australia listed 2,674 elder care homes that offered COVID-19 vaccinations with the majority of the facilities having provided 70–90% of the primary injections and the first booster to their residents. The other percentages for these facilities were as follows: 73 of the service providers only completed a 60% vaccination rate; three elder care providers gave 40% of their residents the COVID vaccine, a 50% immunization rate was provided in 35 of the facilities listed, and a 30% vaccination rate was identified in another six elder care provider facilities.[35]

Spain

A Spanish study estimated that COVID infections and deaths were reduced by three-quarters once 70% of LTC residents were fully vaccinated.[36] This particular 17-study analysis also revealed that some of the evaluations did not have such positive results in their analysis and felt that HCW vaccination was a contributing factor to the lack of decline in resident COVID infection rates.

Improvement in vaccinations for future pandemics

In the United States, obtaining COVID vaccinations for the gerontological client and employees was not a problematic situation on any level, a problem did develop with regard to obtaining consent for the vaccination administration process. There were refusals obtained from residents, employees, and resident representatives; with the majority of concerns being related to the individuals feeling the vaccines were developed too quickly and there was no knowledge of definitive potential side effects from the vaccines. Even with additional education provided to potential recipients of the vaccines, the refusals remained sustained in most cases.

For future pandemics, the CDC has released education on building vaccine confidence that addresses a belief supporting that vaccines work, are safe, and are part of a trustworthy medical system. It is further elaborated on that vaccine decision-making is based on cultural, social, and political factors; individual and group factors; and vaccine-specific factors. The WHO implemented a three Cs model of confidence, complacency, and convenience:

• Boost Confidence in Safety and effectiveness of COVID-19 vaccines
• Combat complacency about the pandemic
• Increase the convenience of getting vaccinated

An analysis with regard to COVID-19 vaccinations that examined 23 countries revealed that 66.4% of the world's population had received at least one dose of the COVID-19 vaccine, but only 17.4% of people in low-income countries had received a first dose, underscoring unequal access, availability, and delivery, which impacted gerontological clients in these countries.[37]

WHO reported that globally 64% (January 2023) of the world's population has been COVID vaccinated with the primary series, but significant disparities existed: Australia stated that only 29% of individuals had been vaccinated, Africa reported that 27% of their population completed the primary series, European countries consisted of a 64% vaccinated rate according to WHO data, and Eastern Mediterranean countries were at a 48% vaccination rate.[38]

Another report, *The Future of Epidemic and Pandemic Vaccines to Serve Global Public Health* released in 2023, revealed that the key to the future epidemic and pandemic responses would be sustainable global public health-driven vaccine development and manufacturing based on equitable access to platform technologies, decentralized and localized innovation, and multiple developers and manufacturers, especially in low- and middle-income countries.[39]

Extensive mitigation strategies were implemented in a lot of LTC facilities globally, yet despite the IPC efforts, COVID-19 cases still occurred. Another article that evaluated 17 studies on COVID-19 vaccine effectiveness including England and Denmark estimated a 60% vaccine effectiveness against infection or higher, after the first dose was administered, and in the United States, they found significantly lower rates of new infections among LTC residents in the few weeks following the start of vaccination drives compared with what would be expected without vaccinations.[40]

In this chapter, we examined mitigation, surveillance, and IPC protocols in nursing homes, and provided suggestions on ways to improve these processes for future pandemics. As an industry, LTC is an ever-evolving system that faces many challenges in the provision of healthcare to the gerontological client but continues to assess and re-evaluate itself in an attempt to improve services.

Notes

1 Andrejko, K. L., et al. (2022). Effectiveness of Face Mask or Respirator Use in Indoor Public Settings for Prevention of SARS-CoV-2 infection. *MMWR Morbidity and Mortality Weekly Report*. Centers for Disease Control and Prevention. 71. https://dx.doi.org/10.15585/mmwr.mm7106e1. (accessed October 17, 2022). pp. 212–216.

2 Wending, Jean-Michel, et al. (2021). Experimental efficiency of the face shield and the mask against emitted and potentially received particles. *International Journal of Environmental Research and Public Health*. 18(4). https://pubmed.ncbi.nlm.nih.gov/33671300/. (accessed October 30, 2022). p. 1942.

3 Parotto, Emanuela, et al. (2023). Exploring Italian healthcare facilities response to COVID-19 pandemic: Lessons learned from the Italian Response to COVID-19 initiative. *Frontiers in Public Health*. 10. https://doi.org/10.3389/fpubh.2022.1016649. (accessed November 3, 2023).

4 Wallenburg, Iris, et al. (2021). Unmasking a healthcare system: The Dutch policy response to the COVOD-19 crisis. *Health Economics, Policy and Law*. 17(1). https://www.cambridge.org/core/journals/health-economics-policy-and-law/article/unmasking-a-health-care-system-the-dutch-policy-response-to-the-covid19-crisis/805887E8BC039AAD89641158 4FF3. (accessed November 3, 2023). pp. 27–36.

5 Dow, William, PhD, et al. (2020). Economic and health benefits of PPE stockpile. *Berkley Public Health*. https://laborcenter.berkeley.edu/wp-content/uploads/2020/08/Economic-Health-Benefits-of-PPE-Stockpile-UC-Berkeley-2020-FINAL.pdf. (accessed July 3, 2023).

6 Best, Stephanie, and Williams, Sharon. (2021). What have we learnt about the sourcing of personal protective equipment during pandemics? Leadership and management in healthcare supply chain management: A scoping review. *Frontiers in Public Health*. 9. www.ncbi.nlm.nih.gov/pmc/articles/PMC8695796/. (accessed July 3, 2023). p. 765501

7 Best, Stephanie, and Williams, Sharon. (2021). What have we learnt about the sourcing of personal protective equipment during pandemics? Leadership and management in healthcare supply chain management: A scoping review. *Frontiers in Public Health*. 9. www.ncbi.nlm.nih.gov/pmc/articles/PMC8695796/. (accessed July 3, 2023). p. 765501

8 Best, Stephanie, and Williams, Sharon. (2021). What have we learnt about the sourcing of personal protective equipment during pandemics? Leadership and management in healthcare supply chain management: A scoping review. *Frontiers in Public Health*. 9. www.ncbi.nlm.nih.gov/pmc/articles/PMC8695796/. (accessed July 3, 2023). p. 765501.

9 Best, Stephanie, and Williams, Sharon. (2021). What have we learnt about the sourcing of personal protective equipment during pandemics? Leadership and management in healthcare supply chain management: A scoping review. *Frontiers in Public Health.* 9. www.ncbi.nlm.nih.gov/pmc/articles/PMC8695796/. (accessed July 3, 2023). p. 765501

10 Best, Stephanie, and Williams, Sharon. (2021). What have we learnt about the sourcing of personal protective equipment during pandemics? Leadership and management in healthcare supply chain management: A scoping review. *Frontiers in Public Health.* 9. www.ncbi.nlm.nih.gov/pmc/articles/PMC8695796/. (accessed July 3, 2023). p. 765501.

11 Cabinet Secretary for NHS Recovery, Health and Social Care. (2022). *Personal Protective Equipment-future Supply: Consultation Analysis.* Scottish Government. www.gov.scot/publications/consultation-future-supply-pandemic-personal-protective-equipment-scotland-analysis-consultation-responses/pages/4/. (accessed July 3, 2023).

12 Cabinet Secretary for NHS Recovery, Health and Social Care. (2022). *Personal Protective Equipment-future Supply: Consultation Analysis.* Scottish Government. www.gov.scot/publications/consultation-future-supply-pandemic-personal-protective-equipment-scotland-analysis-consultation-responses/pages/4/. (accessed July 3, 2023).

13 Cabinet Secretary for NHS Recovery, Health and Social Care. (2022). *Personal Protective Equipment-future Supply: Consultation Analysis.* Scottish Government. www.gov.scot/publications/consultation-future-supply-pandemic-personal-protective-equipment-scotland-analysis-consultation-responses/pages/4/. (accessed July 3, 2023).

14 Centers for Disease Control and Prevention. (2023). Infection control assessment and response (ICAR) tool for general infection prevention and control (IPAC) across settings. www.cdc.gov/hai/prevent/infection-control-assessment-tools.html. (accessed July 4, 2023).

15 Clinical Excellence Commission. (2023). *Infection Prevention and Control Manual COVID-19 and Other Acute Respiratory Infections for Acute and Non-acute Healthcare Settings*, v4.1. Sydney, Australia: Clinical Excellence Commission. https://www.cec.health.nsw.gov.au/__data/assets/pdf_file/0018/644004/IPAC-Manual-COVID-19-and-Other-ARIs-version-4.1-280623.pdf. (accessed July 4, 2023).

16 National Health Service England. (2023). National infection prevention and control manual for England. www.england.nhs.uk/wp-content/uploads/2022/04/PRN00123-national-infection-prevention-and-control-manual-for-england-v2.5.pdf. (accessed July 4, 2023).

17 Ireton, Julie. (2021). Rapid testing will add to strain on long-term care sector, advocates warn. www.cbc.ca/news/canada/ottawa/rapid-testing-concerns-long-term-care-added-pressure-staffing-1.5912517. (accessed October 25, 2022).

18 Salmeron, Sergio, et al. (2022). Efficiency of diagnostic test for SARS-CoV-2 in a nursing home. *Geriatrics.* 7(4). https://doi.org/10.3390/geriatrics7040078. (accessed October 29, 2022). p. 78.

19 Salmeron, Sergio, et al. (2022). Efficiency of diagnostic test for SARS-CoV-2 in a nursing home. *Geriatrics.* 7(4). https://doi.org/10.3390/geriatrics7040078. (accessed October 29, 2022). p. 78.

20 Savio, Antonella, et al. (2021). Rapid point-of-care serology and clinical history nursing homes in Brescia, a hotspot of Lombardy. *Frontiers.* 9:1–9. https://doi.org/10.3389/pubh.2021.649524. (accessed October 29, 2022).

21 National Institute for Public Health and the Environment, Ministry of Health, Welfare and Sport. (2020). Policy on testing for novel coronavirus disease (COVID-19). www.rivm.nl/en/novel-coronavirus-covid-19/testing-policy. (accessed November 3, 2023).

22 Centers for Medicare & Medicaid Services. (2022). COVID-19 nursing home data. https://data.cms.gov/covid-19/covid-19-nursing-home-data. (accessed October 30, 2022).

23 Centers for Medicare & Medicaid Services. (2020). Trump Administration has issued more than $15 million in fines to nursing homes during COVID-19 pandemic. https://cms.gov/newsroom/press-releases/trump-administration-has-issued-more-15-million-fines-to-nursing-homes-during-covid-19-pandemic. (accessed October 23, 2022).

24 Centers for Medicare & Medicaid Services. (2022). COVID-19 nursing home data. https://data.cms.gov/covid-19/covid-19-nursing-home-data. (accessed October 30, 2022).

25 Centers for Medicare & Medicaid Services. (2022). COVID-19 nursing home data. https://data.cms.gov/covid-19/covid-19-nursing-home-data. (accessed October 30, 2022).

26 Centers for Medicare & Medicaid Services. (2022). COVID-19 nursing home data. https://data.cms.gov/covid-19/covid-19-nursing-home-data. (accessed October 30, 2022).

27 Centers for Disease Control and Prevention. (2023). COVID-19 nursing home data. https://data.cms.gov/covid-19/covid-19-nursing-home-data. (accessed October 1, 2023).

28 Centers for Disease Control and Prevention. (2023). COVID-19 nursing home data. https://data.cms.gov/covid-19/covid-19-nursing-home-data. (accessed October 1, 2023).

29 Centers for Disease Control and Prevention. (2023). COVID-19 nursing home data. Center for Medicare and Medicaid Services. https://data.cms.gov/covid-19/covid-19-nursing-home-data. (accessed May 12, 2023).

30 Comas-Herrera. (2021). The rollout of COVID-19 vaccines in Canadian long-term care homes, 9th April update. https://ltccovid.org/2021/04/12/the-rollout-of-covid-19-vaccines-long-term-care-homes-9th-april-update/amp/. (accessed October 30, 2022).

31 Brown, Kevin, et al. (2021). Early impact of Ontario's COVID-19 vaccine rollout on long-term care home residents and health care workers. *Science Briefs of the Ontario COVID-19 Advisory Table.* 2(13). https://doi.org/10.47326/ocsat.2021.02.13.1.0. (accessed October 30, 2022).

32 Paola, Frati, et al. (2021). Compulsory vaccination for healthcare workers in Italy for the prevention of SARS-CoV-2 infection. *Vaccines (Basel).* 9(9). https://doi.org/10.3390/vaccines9090966. https://pubmed.ncbi.nlm.nih.gov/34579203/. (accessed November 3, 2023). p. 966.

33 Rivasi, Giulia, et al. (2021). Course and lethality of SARS-CoV-2 in nursing homes after vaccination in Florence, Italy. *Vaccines.* 9(10). https://doi.org/10.3390/vaccines9101174. (accessed October 30, 2022). p. 1174.

34 BBC News. (2021). Covid care home vaccine 'milestone' reached in England. www.com/news/uk-55881741.amp. (accessed October 30, 2022).
35 Australian Government Department of Health and Aged Care. (2022). Residential aged care residents COVID-19 vaccination rates. www.health. gov.au/initiatives-and-programs/covid-19-vaccination/information-for-aged-care-providers-workers-and-residents-about-covid-19-vaccines/residential-aged-care-residents. (accessed October 30, 2022).
36 Salcher-Konrad, Maximilian, et al. (2021). Emerging evidence on effectiveness of COVID-19 vaccines among residents of long-term care facilities. *Journal of the American Medical Directors Association.* 22(8). www.ncbi.nlm.nih.gov/pmc/articles/PMC148429. (accessed October 30, 2022). pp. 1602, 1603.
37 Lazarus, Jeffery, et al. (2023). A survey of COVID-19 vaccine acceptance across 23 countries in 2022. *Nature Medicine.* 29. https://doi.org/10.1038/s41591-022-02185-4. (accessed October 3, 2023). pp. 366–375.
38 World Health Organization. (2023). Update on global COVID-19 vaccination. *Member State Briefing.* https://apps.who.int/gb/COVID-19/pdf_files/2023/05_01/Item1.pdf. (accessed May 12, 2023).
39 Farlow, Andrew, et al. (2023). The future of epidemic and pandemic vaccines to serve global public health needs. *Vaccines.* 11(3). https://doi.org/10.3390/vaccines11030690. (accessed October 3, 2023). p. 690.
40 Salcher-Konrad, Maximilian, et al. (2021). Emerging evidence on effectiveness of COVID-19 vaccines among residents of long-term care facilities. *Journal of the American Medical Directors Association.* 22(8). www.ncbi.nlm.nih.gov/pmc/articles/PMC148429. (accessed October 30, 2022). pp. 1602–1603.

4 Public Health Emergency
Termination and Policy Changes

The Biden Administration announced on January 30, 2023, that the National PHE would end on May 11, 2023, in the United States. The Emergency Committee of the Pan American Health Department advised the WHO Director-General on May 5, 2023, to transition to long-term management of the COVID-19 pandemic, as it no longer constituted a PHE of international concern, due to continued decreases in deaths, positive cases identified, and hospitalizations.

Through discussion of current statistics, the many different variants of COVID that have emerged worldwide, and the PHE Termination protocols regarding testing, vaccination, reporting, EUA, waivers, and IPC policies (including recommendations by WHO and the CDC), there can be improved knowledge for future pandemics related to policies, protocols, and procedures.

In 2023, coronavirus outbreaks in nursing homes still existed globally, but they were not as frequent or lethal as at the beginning of the pandemic. Some epidemiologists and infection control experts believe that COVID-19 may become a seasonal illness with predictable patterns of infection, but it is not there yet; it could take a few more years to achieve this status as herd immunity is achieved.

2023 Global Statistics

In the period from March 13 to April 9, 2023, there were three million new cases of COVID-19 and its variants diagnosed, and 23,000 deaths reported worldwide.[1] Also, in the 28-day period from July 31 to August 27, 2023, over 1.4 million new COVID-19 cases and over 1,800 deaths were reported to WHO.[2] Globally, positive COVID cases and deaths are still occurring today. Figure 4.1 illustrates a breakdown of the globally reported COVID cases during a 30-day period in 2023.

The United States

In the United States, the average daily COVID hospital admission rate on May 12, 2023, was 4,275 people, the average positivity test rate was 5.3% on

DOI: 10.4324/9781003466192-7

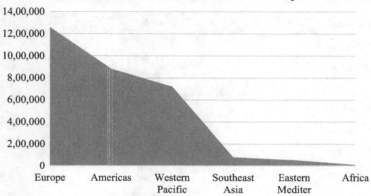

Figure 4.1 New Global Cases of COVID in 30 Days in 2023.[3]

Source: The New York Times. This is an area graph with a vertical axis of numbers from 200,000 to 1,400,000 and a horizontal axis of global regions, showing the number of new COVID cases in 30 days (2023), with Africa having the lowest number at 9,155 positive cases and Europe at the highest with 1,257,642 new cases.

May 7, 2023, and the primary series national completion vaccination rate was at 69%.[4] Figure 4.2 depicts the number of positive COVID cases identified in specific US states during the week of April 27 to May 3, 2023.

US nursing homes had 5,462 confirmed positive resident COVID cases identified in the week ending 4/16/2023 and 132 resident deaths. Also, in the week ending April 30, 2023, there were 2,624 employee positive COVID cases identified and 10 employee deaths.[5] In July and August 2023, SARS-CoV-2 outbreaks were on the rise again in US nursing homes, and it is estimated that there had been 5,000 nursing home residents that died from COVID by October 2023.

Ireland

In Ireland, 191 COVID-19 outbreaks had been reported by February 2023, and key outbreak locations included:

1. 57 (29.8%) were reported in hospitals.
2. 77 (40.3%) were reported in nursing homes.
3. 16 (8.4%) were reported in community hospital/long-stay units.
4. 38 (19.9%) were reported in residential institutions.
5. 2 (1.0%) were reported in "other" healthcare services.
6. 1 (0.5%) were reported in a range of other settings.[7]

US COVID-Positive Cases in One Week in 2023

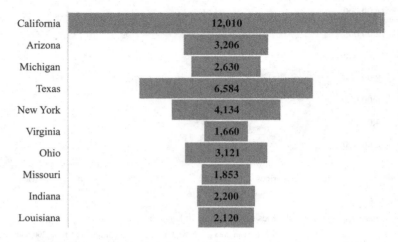

Figure 4.2 Positive COVID Cases in US States in One Week in 2023.[6]

Source: *The New York Times.* This figure illustrates a vertical axis showing specific US states and the number of positive COVID cases in one week, with Virginia at the lowest with 1,660 new cases and California at the highest with 12,010 cases.

England

Coronavirus testing in care homes continues in England. In the week ending January 15, 2023:

- There were 1,522 positive lateral flow test results among care home staff. The number had been decreasing since the week ending January 1, 2023, when 3,702 positive tests were recorded.
- There were 442 positive lateral flow test results among care home residents. This number had been decreasing since the week ending December 25, 2022, when 992 positive tests were recorded.[8]

Switzerland

By the end of January 2023, Switzerland had 7,405 additional positive COVID cases identified in their country including Zurich—1,263 cases, Bern—814 cases, Vaud—813 cases, Geneva—469 cases, and Ticino—802 cases.[9]

SARS-CoV-2 Variants

There have been multiple variants of the SARS-CoV-2 virus that have emerged worldwide. A *variant* is a viral genome (genetic code) that may contain one or more mutations; Alpha and Delta variants were identified first in 2020. Omicron (B.1.1.529) is the COVID virus variant that was reported by South Africa to WHO in November 2021. Figure 4.3 illustrates the number of countries where specific variants of SARS-CoV-2 have emerged in causing infections.

Experts report that the Omicron variant spreads more easily than the original SARS-CoV-2 virus and the Delta variant, but lethality did not appear to be as pronounced. Updated vaccine boosters were bivalent, designed to protect against SARS-CoV-2 (Beta and Delta variants), Omicron, and its variants BA.1–BA.5. Variants of Omicron continue to emerge in 2023, with BQ.1, BQ.11, XBB.1.5, XBB1.16, and XBB1.9.1 being identified in numerous countries.

In May 2023, the original omicron variant was gone; the dominant variants in the United States were XBB.1.5 (64% of the cases), then XBB.1.16 (14.3% of the cases), and XBB.1.9.1 (9.2% of the cases).[11] The plasticity of the virus suggests that more variants are possible, and some could be worse than Omicron. One of the newest strains identified in 2023 is EG.5. By August 7, 2023, 7,354 sequences (virus genetic material) of EG.5 have been submitted to the Global Initiative on Sharing All Influenza Data (GISAID) from 51 countries. The largest portion of EG.5 sequences are from China (30.6%, 2,247

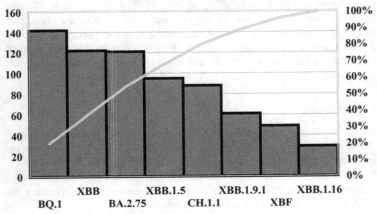

Figure 4.3 SARS-CoV-2 Variants in Different Countries.[10]

Source: World Health Organization. This is a histogram graph that illustrates two vertical axes: one on the right with numbers from 0 to 160 and one on the left with percentages from 0% to 100%, and a horizontal axis with COVID variants listed, showing the number of countries that SARS-CoV-2 variants have emerged, with BQ.1 at above 140 countries and XBB.1.16 noted in around 30 countries.

sequences). The other countries with at least 100 sequences are the United States (18.4%, 1356 sequences), the Republic of Korea (14.1%, 1,040 sequences), Japan (11.1%, 814 sequences), Canada (5.3%, 392 sequences), Australia (2.1%, 158 sequences), Singapore (2.1%, 154 sequences), the United Kingdom (2.0%, 150 sequences), France (1.6%,119 sequences), Portugal (1.6%, 115 sequences), and Spain (1.5%, 107 sequences).[12]

Also, BA.2.86 was first detected in Denmark. On August 17, 2023, the WHO classified BA.2.86 as a variant under monitoring. The new variant, with a range of new spike (S) gene mutations, was quickly detected in several countries, including Israel, South Africa, the United Kingdom, and the United States, suggesting international transmission.[13] Potential risks need to be managed, especially in nursing homes, based on how these viruses might evolve to become more transmissible and potentially more lethal in the future.

PHE Termination: US LTC Policy Changes

When the PHE ended in America on May 11, 2023, nursing homes were still required to report their COVID data to the NHSN CDC on a weekly basis but were no longer having to report positive cases to residents and families. The CDC and CMS utilize this information to strengthen COVID-19 surveillance locally and nationally; to monitor trends in infection rates; and to help local, state, and federal health authorities in providing help to nursing homes.

Nursing homes reporting data to the CDC is a critical component of the national COVID-19 surveillance system. The information is also posted online allowing the public to be aware of how the COVID-19 virus is affecting nursing homes. Failure to report data continues to result in the imposition of a civil money penalty for each occurrence of non-reporting as follows: a civil money penalty of $1,000 for the first occurrence, followed by $500 added to the previously imposed civil money penalty for each subsequent occurrence.

COVID Testing

As far as guidance provided on COVID testing, it was relayed that testing would continue as the standards put forth by the CDC for IPC requirements and is applicable one year beyond the expiration of the PHE for COVID-19. Medicare and Medicaid covered the costs of COVID testing when ordered by a physician, nurse practitioner, or physician's assistant until September 30, 2024, when potential cost sharing was applicable.

COVID Vaccination

In addition, COVID vaccination administrations for residents and staff were mandated to be provided and reported to the CDC "indefinitely" until other directives are given per the CMS. After the end of the PHE, CMS continued to pay approximately $40 per dose for administering COVID-19 vaccines for Medicare/Medicaid beneficiaries in nursing homes. After June 30, 2023, immunizers were no longer able to bill Medicare directly for vaccines furnished to patients for a Medicare Part A-covered SNF stay. On July 1, 2023, typical SNF consolidated billing regulations were put back in place, which required SNFs to bill for all services furnished to patients in a Medicare-covered SNF stay, including vaccines.

Emergency Use Authorization

CMS covers and pays for EUA drugs and biologicals for COVID-19 the same way it covers and pays for COVID-19 vaccines when furnished consistent with the EUA. There is also no beneficiary cost sharing and no deductible for COVID-19 monoclonal antibody products when providers administer them. As these products become approved or authorized for use, they will continue to be covered and paid for; this coverage and payment will continue even after the end of the PHE. CMS does not pay for the COVID-19 monoclonal antibody product if a healthcare setting has received it for free. If a healthcare setting purchases the product from the manufacturer, CMS pays the reasonable cost or 95% of the average wholesale price.

The FDA approved VEKLURYTM (Remdesivir) as a treatment for COVID-19. CMS provides payment for the drug and its administration under the applicable payment policy when a facility or practitioner provides it in the clinical setting. In most cases, the Medicare patient's yearly Part B deductible and 20% co-insurance apply. Beginning on January 1, 2024, for beneficiaries in a Medicare Part A-covered SNF stay, payment for Remdesivir will be subject to SNF consolidated billing and will not be separately billable to Part B.

Waivers

Almost all waivers for nursing homes granted during the PHE expired on May 11, 2023. However, telehealth was still approved for utilization until December 2024. Some examples of provider telehealth in nursing homes are virtual check-ins, brief 5–10-minute e-visits, and remote evaluations conducted through technology mediums. CMS released the Long-Term Care Nursing Home Telehealth and Telemedicine Tool Kit in March 2020 to assist in the continuity of provider services during the pandemic.

PHE Termination: Other Countries, LTC Policy Changes

England released new directives for adult social care in April 2023, that recommended symptomatic testing only for those eligible for COVID-19 treatments and during suspected outbreaks, and positively tested individuals could return to usual activities after five days if displaying no high temperature. Also, during an outbreak, only the first five residents would be tested with the lateral flow device (LFD, used for asymptomatic testing) test, and outbreak measures could be lifted five days past the last confirmed case. All restrictions on visitation for asymptomatic/non-positive residents had been terminated. In addition, all new admissions will have an LFD test conducted within 48 hours of discharge from the hospital, and COVID vaccination processes would be ongoing.[14]

Canada

Changed guidance in Ontario, Canada's IPC practices for care homes was given in March 2023 and established the discontinuation of screening protocols, physical distancing, and outdoor masking. It was advised that daily temperature checks were only to be conducted for residents who were positive or symptomatic and that COVID testing would only be conducted on symptomatic residents.[15]

Australia

Australia in April 2023 updated recommendations for LTC facilities that entailed the following information: For the best protection, the expert Australian Technical Advisory Group on Immunization (ATAGI) recommends an early 2023 COVID-19 vaccine booster dose for adults aged 18 years or older if their last COVID-19 vaccine dose or confirmed infection (whichever is the most recent) was six months ago or longer, and regardless of the number of prior doses received.[16]

Lagevrio (molnupiravir) and Paxlovid (nirmatrelvir plus ritonavir) are two oral antiviral medicines that may help stop a COVID-19 infection from becoming severe. Both treatments have been shown to reduce the chance of a person needing admission to the hospital for treatment and severe illness. All Australians aged 70 years or over who test COVID-19 positive, with or without symptoms can access these oral antivirals on the Pharmaceutical Benefits Scheme (PBS). Also eligible for Paxlovid are people aged 60–69 years with one risk factor, and people over 50 years with two risk factors for developing severe disease.[17]

In addition, it was recommended that residential aged care homes actively screen for symptoms of COVID-19 in residents being admitted or re-admitted from other health facilities and community settings. And, visitors to residential aged care who have tested positive for COVID-19 must not visit high-risk settings like residential aged care homes for at least seven days after testing positive and until they have no symptoms of COVID-19.[18]

Ireland

An article (2023) in the *Irish Times* stated that HCWs were no longer required to wear face masks for all interactions with patients in nursing homes and other residential care facilities.

New HSE COVID-19 guidance stated that staff should continue to wear high-grade masks when dealing with infectious patients or where there is a high risk of undiagnosed cases being present. The guidelines emphasized that social activity was an essential part of community life in care facilities and should no longer be limited on infection control grounds, other than when a resident is infectious or an outbreak needs to be managed.[19]

Scotland

In May 2023, Scotland updated their guidelines stating that continuous use of face masks in social care settings, including care homes, was no longer required nor advised routinely. This was due to the effective combination of natural and vaccine immunity in protecting populations at this stage of the pandemic and the risks that covering the face can present to social interaction, particularly for vulnerable individuals.

Vaccination of staff and service users, particularly in care homes, had altered the COVID-19 mitigation measures, making systems less restrictive—for both vaccinated and unvaccinated people. Where possible, staff and service users should be assessed for vaccine status and offered COVID-19 (and other) vaccinations at the earliest opportunity.

Physical distancing was no longer required for staff, service users, or visitors. Some health and social care services may choose to continue with physical distancing measures, in particular, if there is a risk of overcrowding.

Testing was no longer mandatory for individuals or staff. The main purpose of COVID-19 testing changed from population-wide testing to reduce transmission to targeted testing to support clinical care, identifying an outbreak as two linked cases of COVID-19 over a 14-day period within a defined setting. COVID-19 outbreak management would continue to follow existing, well-established public health principles and practices.[20]

World Health Organization

WHO provided pandemic guidance in March 2023, based on situational levels in countries including:

- Situational Level 1: Minimal transmission, morbidity, and health system impact of SARS-CoV-2, with only basic ongoing public health and social measures (PHSM) needed. Ensure support for institutional isolation of infected individuals. Health service infrastructure, bed capacity, and patient flow are to be assessed for anticipated limitations and contingency measures to continue essential operations in the event of an unanticipated surge. This includes care of patients in isolation and health services to screen staff, patients, and visitors for signs and symptoms of respiratory infection.[21]

* Situational level 2: Moderate impact of COVID-19, although there may be higher impact in specific sub-populations. Additional PHSM may be required to reduce transmission. However, disruptions to social and economic activities can still be limited, particularly if PHSM can be targeted strategically to more impacted settings. Implement universal use of medical masks for all staff, patients, and visitors. Continue to assess for capacity and contingency measures to maintain care operations in the event of an unanticipated surge, including care of patients in isolation. Institute surveillance and monitoring for clusters and transmission.[22]

CDC Guidance

Again, May 11, 2023, marked the end of the federal COVID-19 PHE declaration. After this date, CDC's authorizations to collect certain types of public health data expired. Monitoring the impact of COVID-19 and the effectiveness of prevention and control strategies remains a public health priority. With the COVID-19 PHE declaration ending, some metrics remained the same, but some changed in frequency, source, or availability. CDC continues to provide sustainable, high-impact, and timely information to inform COVID decision-making.

The reporting of COVID-19 deaths continues, but the source of data collection changed to the National Vital Statistics System (NVSS), which is the most accurate and complete source of death data, and timeliness of death certificate reporting that has improved over the course of the pandemic. The addition of a new metric, the percent of deaths that are COVID-19-associated is being utilized, and other metrics from NVSS are reported weekly.[23]

COVID-19 positivity test reporting remains in place, but the source of data changed: After May 25, 2023 CDC reports regional-level test positivity data from the National Respiratory and Enteric Virus Surveillance System (NREVSS), a long-standing system with over 450 labs from across the country that voluntarily submit data. These data can provide early indications of COVID-19 transmission.[24]

Counts of COVID-19 vaccines administered remain in place for jurisdictions that continue to submit data, but the frequency changed. This data is updated monthly, instead of weekly.[25] To continue facilitating access to national COVID-19 surveillance data, a first-phase, redesigned COVID Data Tracker website was launched on May 11, 2023. These ongoing data collections will continue providing an evidence base of information to guide prioritization of public health action.

The termination of the PHE instituted many changes in LTC provisions related to SARS-CoV-2. Many different variants have emerged, and the continued transmission of COVID in nursing homes remains to elicit challenges and lessons learned that establish ongoing system evaluations and mitigation implementations in this industry. Reforms in protocols for a PHE termination could potentially encompass one universal set of policies and procedures for the LTC industry, as there was variance between states in the United States, and between countries regarding implemented or terminated protocols and practices. The WHO, CDC, and ECDC contributed immensely to the global PHE mitigation and should be acknowledged for all the efforts they provided over the course of the COVID-19 pandemic.[20]

Notes

1 World Health Organization. (2023). Weekly epidemiological update on COVID-19–13 April 2023. www.who.int/publications/m/item/weekly-epidemiological-update-on-covid-19–13-april-2023. (accessed May 12, 2023).

2 World Health Organization. (2023). Weekly epidemiological update on COVID-19–1 September 2023. www.who.int/publications/m/item/weekly-epidemiological-update-on-covid-19–1-september-2023. (accessed October 3, 2023).

3 The New York Times. (2023). Track COVID-19 in the US. Centers for Disease Control and Prevention. www.nytimes.com/interactive/2023/us/covid-cases.html. (accessed May 12, 2023).

4 World Health Organization. (2023). Weekly epidemiological update on COVID-19–13 April 2023. www.who.int/publications/m/item/weekly-epidemiological-update-on-covid-19–13-april-2023. (accessed May 12, 2023).

5 Centers for Disease Control and Prevention. (2023). COVID-19 nursing home data. Centers for Medicare & Medicaid Services. https://data.cms.gov/covid-19/covid-19-nursing-home-data. (accessed May 12, 2023).

6 The New York Times. (2023). Track COVID-19 in the US. Centers for Disease Control and Prevention. www.nytimes.com/interactive/2023/us/covid-cases.html. (accessed May 12, 2023).

7 Health Protection Surveillance Centre. (2023). Epidemiology of COVID-19 outbreaks/clusters in Ireland – Weekly report. *Week 6*. www.hpsc.ie/a-z/respiratory/coronavirus/novelcoronavirus/surveillance/covid-19outbreaksclustersin ireland/covid-19outbreaksclustersinirelandweeklyreports2023/ Weekly_COVID-19_Outbreak_Report_Week_06_2023_Web_final.pdf.(accessed May 13, 2023).

8 Department of Health and Social Care. (2023). Adult social care monthly statistics England, February 2023. https://www.gov.uk/government/statistics/adult-social-care-in-england-monthly-statistics-february-2023/ adult-social-care-monthly-statistics-england-february-2023. (accessed May 13, 2023).

9 Statista. (2023). Number of confirmed coronavirus (COVID-19) cases in Switzerland in 2023, by canton. www.statista.com/statistics/1107224/coronavirus-covid-19-switzerland-by-canton/. (accessed May 13, 2023).

10 World Health Organization. (2023). Weekly epidemiological update on COVID-19–13 April 2023. www.who.int/publications/m/item/weekly-epidemiological-update-on-covid-19–13-april-2023. (accessed May 12, 2023).

11 Nebraska Medicine. (2023). What COVID-19 variants are going around in May 2023? University of Nebraska Medical Center. www.nebraskamed.com/COVID/what-covid-19-variants-are-going-around. (accessed May 20, 2023).

12 World Health Organization. (2023). EG.5 initial risk evaluation, 9 August 2023. https://www.who.int/docs/default-source/coronaviruse/09082023eg.5_ire_final.pdf?sfvrsn=2aa2daee_1. (accessed November 4, 2023).

13 Morten, Rasmussen, et al. (2023). First cases of SARS-CoV-2 BA.2.86 in Denmark. *Euro Surveill.* 0013;28(36). https://doi.org/10.2807/1560-7917.ES.2023.28.36.2300460. (accessed November 4, 2023).

14 Department of Health and Social Care. (2023). Guidance-COVID-19 supplement to the infection prevention and control source for adult social care. https://ww.gov.uk/government/publications/infection-prevention-and-control-in-adult-social-care-covid-19-supplement/covid-19-supplement-to-the-infection-prevention-and-control-resource-for-adult-social-care. (accessed May 23, 2023).

15 Ministry of Health. (2023). COVID-19 guidance: Long-term care homes, retirement homes, and other congregate living settings for public health units. www.health.gov.on.ca/en/pro/programs/publichealth/coronavirus/docs/LTCH_RH_guidance_PHU.pdf. (accessed May 23, 2023).

16 Australian Government, Department of Health and Aged Care. (2023). COVID-19 advice for people in residential aged care home and visitors. www.health.gov.au/topics/aged-care/advice-on-aged-care-during-covid-19/covid-19-advice-for-people-in-residential-aged-care-home-and-visitors. (accessed May 23, 2023).

17 Australian Government, Department of Health and Aged Care. (2023). COVID-19 advice for people in residential aged care home and visitors. www.health.gov.au/topics/aged-care/advice-on-aged-care-during-covid-19/covid-19-advice-for-people-in-residential-aged-care-home-and-visitors. (accessed May 23, 2023).

18 Australian Government, Department of Health and Aged Car. (2023). COVID-19 advice for people in residential aged care home and visitors. www.health.gov.au/topics/aged-care/advice-on-aged-care-during-covid-19/covid-19-advice-for-people-in-residential-aged-care-home-and-visitors. (accessed May 23, 2023).

19 Cullen, Paul. (2023). COVID-19: Universal mask requirement for nursing home staff removed. *The Irish Times.* https://www.irishtimes.com/health/2023/04/05/covid-19-universal-mask-requirement-for-nursing-home-staff-removed/. (accessed May 29, 2023).

20 Public Health Scotland. (2023). COVID-19 information and guidance for social, community, and residential care settings, Version 2.7

May 2023. https://publichealthscotland.scot/publication s/covid-19-information-and-guidance-for-social-community-and-residential-care-settings/covid-19-information-and-guidance-for-social-community-and-residential-care-settings-version-27/#section-9. (accessed May 29, 2023).

21 World Health Organization. (2023). Considerations for implementing and adjusting public health and social measures in the context of COVID-19. www.who.int/publications/i/item/who-2019-ncov-adjusting-ph-measures-2023.1. (accessed May 23, 2023).

22 World Health Organization. (2023). Considerations for implementing and adjusting public health and social measures in the context of COVID-19. www.who.int/publications/i/item/who-2019-ncov-adjusting-ph-measures-2023.1. (accessed May 23, 2023).

23 Centers for Disease Control and Prevention. (2023). End of the federal COVID-19 Public Health Emergency (PHE) declaration. National Center for Immunization and Respiratory Diseases (NCIRD), Division of Viral Diseases. https://www.cdc.gov/coronavirus/2019-ncov/your-health/end-of-phe.html. (accessed May 29, 2023).

24 Centers for Disease Control and Prevention. (2023). End of the federal COVID-19 Public Health Emergency (PHE) declaration. National Center for Immunization and Respiratory Diseases (NCIRD), Division of Viral Diseases. https://www.cdc.gov/coronavirus/2019-ncov/your-health/end-of-phe.html. (accessed May 29, 2023).

25 Centers for Disease Control and Prevention. (2023). End of the federal COVID-19 Public Health Emergency (PHE) declaration. National Center for Immunization and Respiratory Diseases (NCIRD), Division of Viral Diseases. https://www.cdc.gov/coronavirus/2019-ncov/your-health/end-of-phe.html. (accessed May 29, 2023).

5 LTC Structural and Internal Changes for Elder Care Provisions

There are many strategies that can be implemented to improve the LTC industry for future pandemics including, increased staffing through retention strategies and higher wages, an enhanced provision of mental healthcare services, building on strategies that support deinstitutionalization, harnessing advocates for LTC residents, and exploring alternatives for financing of new LTC facility construction.

Additionally, the LTC facility architecture needs to be redesigned for the provision of effective social distancing, to enhance accommodations for isolation, and in ways to decrease the potential for transmission of infections from the community into a facility, improving resilience. By restructuring elder care living environments to a model that is better equipped to deter pandemic adversities, we could decrease morbidity and mortality with the next pandemic. There are several avenues to examine with restructuring of LTC facilities, such as revisions to current standing facilities, greenhouses, construction of new nursing homes with fewer beds, and the clustered neighborhood designs.

Redesigning LTC Facilities

Revisions to Currently Constructed LTC Facilities

Several different avenues can be evaluated when assessing revision potentials in nursing homes. One would be decreasing the number of beds in each room, converting a four-bedroom room into a two-bedroom room and a two-bedroom room into a single occupancy room. This would allow for more effective social distancing and implementation of isolation protocols in elder care environments within existing facilities.

In addition, instead of utilizing large dining rooms and activity spaces in current care homes, institute small neighborhood spaces utilizing nooks and crannies in facilities to serve fewer patients, yet still allowing for psychosocial needs to be met, and social distancing to be maintained. Additionally, during pandemics, allowing for increased utilization of outdoor spaces with social

DOI: 10.4324/9781003466192-8

distancing could assist in preventing a decline in the residents' mental and emotional health.

The development of Red Isolation Units in nursing homes is another process that requires evaluation and restructuring. As previously stated, the architectural design of some facilities does not allow for a separate entrance and exit that is safe. The construction of new additions or extensions to existing buildings would enhance safe isolative practices and additions to these facilities could also potentially be considered for clustered room designs, also.

Clustered Room Designs

Many countries have instituted the clustered room design model for LTC; within each cluster, there is a living room, dining room, kitchen, outdoor space, and single occupancy rooms. There are usually 8–12 private rooms for each neighborhood cluster.

A study of 17 RACF in four Australian states providing a clustered room design model revealed that homelike, clustered domestic models of elder care are associated with better direct care hours and staff education.[1] Another option similar to the clustered room design is Green Houses.

Green Houses

The Green House Project in the United States, developed by Dr. William Thomas, provides for gerontological clients to be cared for in a non-institutionalized home environment. The program itself assists companies and individuals to build or convert residential homes for elder care.

Typically, Green Houses are perceived as a "household model" with under 20 beds that provide autonomy, green living, intimacy, smart technology, and warmth. There are currently 359 Green House homes in 32 American states, with the majority being licensed skilled nursing facilities in communities that have demonstrated to:

- Have lower rates of COVID infections and deaths
- Better staffing ratios
- Higher occupancy rates
- Superior quality of life for elders

A team at the University of North Carolina's (UNC's) Program on Aging, Disability, and Long-Term Care found that "Green House" residents were far less likely to be infected and to die from a viral transmission than residents of traditional nursing homes.

"There is something beneficial about small nursing homes and Green House homes in particular when it comes to COVID," says Sheryl Zimmerman, a UNC professor who codirects the aging program.[2]

Long before COVID-19 cast a spotlight on nursing homes, researchers who study aging viewed Green Houses as a uniquely human form of housing and care for vulnerable elders that provide a better quality of life while reducing hospital admissions, Medicare spending, and staff turnover.[3]

Additionally, the construction of new LTC facilities could encompass the Green House or Clustered Room design models.

Building New LTC Facilities

Worldwide, governments need to examine the concept of construction of new LTC facilities. In the United States, life safety code standards could be revisited and new standards implemented through CMS specifying that all newly constructed LTC facilities should be 60 beds or under and have single occupancy rooms with their own restroom and shower availability. And, Congress could assess Medicare and Medicaid participation standards for LTC, requiring smaller model homes, thus assisting in the phasing out of larger nursing homes.

Architectural designs of nursing homes have significant impacts on COVID-19 transmissions in elder care settings. Considering the vulnerability of LTC residents in congregated living environments, nursing homes will continue to be high-risk areas for infection outbreaks. To improve the safety and resilience of LTC facilities against future public health emergencies—facility guidelines, financing, and regulations need to be restructured to accommodate an increase in private rooms and living areas, especially with all newly constructed facilities.[4]

Financing Construction of New LTC Facilities

In the United States, the Department of Housing and Urban Development (HUD) contains the Office of Healthcare Programs (OHP) that is located within the Office of Housing and administers FHA's (Federal Housing Administration) healthcare programs; Section 232 of the Mortgage Insurance for Residential Care Facilities program enables affordable financing and refinancing of healthcare facility projects nationwide.

The Office of Residential Care Facilities (ORCF) manages the Section 232 program, which provides mortgage insurance for residential care facilities, such as assisted living facilities, nursing homes, intermediate care facilities, and board and care homes. Section 232 may be used to finance the purchase of a new nursing home or to refinance a facility, for a new LTC facility construction, or for a substantial facility rehabilitation project. Also, a combination of these processes is acceptable—for example, refinancing of a nursing home coupled with a new construction of an assisted living facility.

FHA's healthcare programs are integral to HUD's community development mission. By reducing the cost of capital needed by residential care facilities to finance the construction, renovation, acquisition, or refinancing of facilities, these programs improve access to quality healthcare and work to decrease overall healthcare costs.

Canada

In Canada, the Long-Term Care Home Capital Development Funding Policy, 2022, was developed to govern the provision of funding to eligible operators to support and accelerate the development of a new LTC home or beds, or the redevelopment of an existing LTC home or beds to the current design standards for LTC homes.

The government in Ontario, Canada, is increasing its construction funding subsidy to support the cost of developing or redeveloping LTC homes; additional funding will help fast-track the construction of new LTC beds. This additionally supports the government's $6.4 billion commitment to build more than 30,000 new beds by 2028 and provide 28,000 upgraded LTC beds across the province.

Eligible projects that started the construction by August 31, 2023, received an additional construction subsidy of up to $35 per bed, per day, for 25 years. In addition, eligible not-for-profit applicants were able to convert up to $15 of the supplemental funding into a construction grant payable at the start of construction, to increase projects' upfront equity and enable them to secure financing.[5]

The United Kingdom

There are different ways to finance the construction of new nursing homes in the United Kingdom. Local authorities or private pay are the most common funding sources of care in the UK. Healthcare Real Estate Investment Trusts (HC-REITs) have been established to boost the supply of nursing homes, but these initiatives have met contrasting success in different countries. Healthcare REITs' property types include senior living facilities, hospitals, medical office buildings, and skilled nursing facilities.[6]

It is argued that nation-specific processes of nursing home securitization are shaped by the interrelationships between three crucial factors: (1) retirement income, (2) public policies dedicated to long-term institutional care, and (3) the relations between the REITs and care providers themselves. In the United Kingdom, one such example is Target Healthcare REIT; they invest exclusively in modern, well-designed, and purpose-built care homes with generous social and outdoor spaces and ensuite wet rooms for every resident. Another example is Impact REIT which also purchases care homes with long-term leases in place with well-established operators.

Spain

The European Investment Bank (EIB) is helping to improve elderly care in Spain by means of an agreement to finance the construction of 19 new retirement homes. The EU bank is providing Vitalia Home with a loan of €57.5 million to help set up these new centers using the *Homes to live in with gardens* model developed by the Spanish company, which is intended to improve living spaces and care for the elderly. The agreement was signed by EIB Vice-President Emma Navarro and the CEO of Vitalia Home, Chema Cosculluela, and is being backed by the Investment Plan for Europe, also known as the "Juncker Plan."[7]

The new residences will be located in Madrid, Catalonia, Castilla y León, Valencia, and Murcia. In total, this new infrastructure will provide 3,200 new places for residents and more than 500 places for people who only require daycare. The investments will help to implement the innovative *Homes to live in with gardens* residential model, which is focused on integrated people-centered care. With this in mind, the new retirement homes will include co-living units (houses): homely spaces for groups of 15–20 elderly people. Direct access from these houses to terraces or gardens will allow residents to enjoy regular open-air co-living.[8]

Australia

The Australian Government provides capital grants to build or upgrade residential aged care accommodation through the Rural, Regional, and Other Special Needs Building Fund as part of the Aged Care Approvals Round. These grants are allocated in accordance with the Aged Care Act and the Grant Principles, 2014. To be allocated a grant, the approved provider must meet one of the following requirements:

• Be located in a rural, regional, or remote area
• Focus on residential aged care for people from special needs groups or people with low means
• Provide services in a region that needs extra residential aged care services[9]

The amount of capital investment necessary in residential aged care in the future requires careful consideration. In 2019, the Aged Care Financing Authority estimated that the combined total investment for new and rebuilt residential care places over the next decade will be about $55 billion. The average cost of building a new residential aged care bed sits at around $250,000.

RACF need to be suitable for delivering the care necessary for older and frail people. They also need to be designed in ways that support a high quality of life for residents, which research suggests may be achieved through smaller facilities.[10] Additionally, as discussed previously, sufficient staffing ratios to provide adequate elder care in all healthcare settings are a necessity to improve quality of life.

Employee Retention

Retention of LTC employees has been an ongoing problem for nursing homes for decades. In a current study examining staff turnover in the industry, UCLA's Ashvin Gandhi, Huizi Yu-an undergraduate student, and Harvard's David Grabowski assessed uniform payroll data the Centers for Medicare & Medicaid Services began collecting in 2016 and identified turnover rates for roughly 15,600 nursing homes in the United States. Revealing averages, rather than medians, turnovers in nursing homes are high—140.7% for RNs, 114.1% for LPNs, and 129.1% for CNAs.[11]

Certified nursing assistants are essential for the provision of quality of care and spend the most time with residents in LTC facilities. Higher compensation for direct care workers is a necessity to attempt to decrease the 129% turnover rate; we need to advocate for a new baseline wage for certified nursing assistants that better reflects their ongoing contribution to the industry. Beyond wages, retention of CNAs in nursing homes can encompass many other factors including; supervision styles, scheduling availabilities, career development opportunities, culture of a facility, the intrinsic rewards of caregiving, staffing-to-patient ratios, and benefit packages. It is estimated that the expense to replace a CNA in LTC is between $3,000 and $6,000, encompassing both direct and indirect cost factors.[12]

High licensed nurse turnover rates in LTC facilities are also attributed to many elements such as stress levels, lack of career recognition, poor management, feeling over-worked, nurse culture in a facility, inability to deliver high-quality service due to workplace/system issues, and feeling undervalued by society and the workplace. A high nurse turnover rate in LTC decreases effective assessments of residents making it more difficult to detect complications, impacts care management strategies, decreases the effectiveness of a therapeutic nurse/client relationship, and affects the overall health outcomes of residents. The average cost of turnover for a staff nurse is over $46,000, and it generally takes at least three months for organizations to recruit experienced nurses.[13]

Turnover of nursing home administrators is an ongoing dilemma in LTC facilities also. In 2001, the average turnover rate for this position was at 43%.[14] High administrator turnover can create instability within a nursing home, and research has found that it can lead to negative effects on nursing home residents. It is estimated that the average tenure for a nursing home administrator in a facility is one to two years. Nursing home administrators are expected to be on-call 24 hours a day, facilitating burnout, which is a major issue. The American College of Health Care Administration (ACHCA) considers nursing home administrator turnover a major issue and is working to relieve the stressors that many administrators face.

Retention of staff is essential for the LTC industry, having a high employee retention rate shows potential residents, nurses, certified nursing assistants, and potential management employees that a facility maintains a successful, positive work environment. In addition, employee retention can reduce costs; long-term employee retention is critical for keeping operational costs low. Maintaining continuity of staff also improves facility ratings and survey processes, enhances facility morale, and increases staffing/patient ratios; thus improving quality of care.

There are many strategies that can be harnessed to improve staff retention, such as developing a positive culture in the facility environment that is respectful and inclusive for all employees, obtaining feedback from employees on their perception of satisfaction with their position, ensuring adequate staffing to decrease burnout, providing adequate wages and benefits, and setting clear and obtainable expectations for job performances within a facility. Providing adequate staffing ratios can assist in sustaining the mental well-being of gerontological clients.

Improving Provision of Mental Health Services in LTC

Some nursing homes prior to the pandemic had pre-established mental health service contracts; nurse practitioners came into the facilities throughout the pandemic to assess, monitor, and provide mental health support for patients. In some cases, psychotropic medications were ordered or dosage adjustments initiated to assist with resident clinical symptomatology. Telemental health was also utilized in facilities that had pre-contracted processes established prior to the PHE.

Unfortunately, there are regions in the United States where mental health support is not as well-established in LTC, due to lack of professional service availability. In these facilities, there are other potential alternatives to assist with identifying and addressing the mental health impact from a pandemic, such as the administration of depression screening protocols, utilization of primary care providers, and having social services involvement in addressing resident concerns and stress.

Also, many mental health professionals recommend utilizing nonpharmacological interventions for dementia residents and other clients who experience neuropsychological symptoms, such as music therapy, touch therapy, activities, pets, exercise, aromatherapy, and reflexology. It has been established, especially with the elderly, that these therapeutic processes are not only effective for decreasing escalation of behaviors but also healthier due to not introducing additional chemicals into a gerontological client's body system. Furthermore, several organizations across the globe have provided recommendations for the provision of mental healthcare in the LTC industry.

American Geriatrics Society, American Association for Geriatric Psychiatry, and the National Coalition on Mental Health and Aging, in America

Even without a pandemic, the maintenance of the mental health of residents and the provision of mental healthcare is a necessity in the elder care industry. During pandemics, it is essential that mental health screening and telemental health are incorporated into the services provided in nursing homes to adequately assess and identify potential mental health decline.

It is also imperative that frontline staff in LTC facilities who spend the majority of time with gerontological clients are knowledgeable about mental conditions and their management. To address the inadequate preparation of frontline nursing home staff as caregivers for residents with mental conditions, the American Geriatrics Society and the American Association for Geriatric Psychiatry recommend the implementation of training models with demonstrated effectiveness. One successful model is the "train the trainer" approach, in which an outside mental health nurse specialist provides ongoing training and consulting to frontline nursing home staff.

The National Coalition on Mental Health and Aging in America believes that critical strategies to address the current and future shortfall in providers who are trained in geriatrics and mental health include:

1. Exploring incentive programs, including loan repayment programs and increased authorization of graduate medical education payments
2. Expanding required training in geriatrics to LTC nurses and other allied professionals in addressing psychiatric disorders and behavioral symptoms of dementia
3. Developing approaches to increase the number of providers with geriatric mental health training, including early educational awareness of geriatrics as a potential career path; development of multidisciplinary training in aging and mental health; increasing provider competencies through information-technology mechanisms; and increasing the proportion of educational programs with training in late-life mental health disorders.[15]

The coalition further states that it is critically important to address workforce shortages in rural and other underserved areas by incentivizing behavioral health providers to practice in these areas.

Another issue that needs to be addressed with regard to future pandemics is who is considered to be an essential worker. It has been reported that some mental health clinicians who were providing behavioral health services to LTC residents began to encounter difficulties when attempting to see their patients; mental health clinicians were refused entry into some LTC facilities, and this disrupted their ability to provide mental health care. And, even if telemental health was utilized in LTC, some psychologists and mental health nurse practitioners have relayed that facilities encountered difficulties, due to a lack of access to available technology and/or finding available staff who could assist with telemental health care delivery.

Canadian Academy of Geriatric Psychiatry and Canadian Coalition for Seniors Mental Health

The Canadian Academy of Geriatric Psychiatry (CAGP) and Canadian Coalition for Seniors Mental Health (CCSMH) developed position statements on mental health care for older adults in LTC during the pandemic, including:

- Mental health care in LTC settings is an essential service.
- Restrictions on in-person visits to LTC must include measures that address the potential negative effects of these restrictions on the mental health, quality of life, and dignity of LTC residents and their families.
- Appropriate communication technology and human resources must be available to allow communications between LTC residents and individuals located outside a resident's LTC facility.
- All LTC facilities must have adequate training, staffing, and resources to assess and treat common mental health conditions during COVID-19 and other infectious disease outbreaks.
- Measures of mental health and quality of life in LTC facilities must be systematically evaluated during COVID-19, and strategies must be implemented to understand and remediate adverse mental health outcomes when they are identified.[16]

The United Nations

The United Nations issued an executive summary that addressed the mental health of individuals during the COVID PHE to assist in minimizing impacts countries need to:

> (1) Apply a whole of society approach to promote, protect, and care for mental health; (2) Ensure widespread availability of emergency mental health and psychosocial support; and (3) Support recovery from COVID-19 by building mental health services for the future.[17]

In the position paper, the United Nations addresses the continuing need for improved mental health services within the community setting for all countries and acknowledges the mental health impacts of a pandemic on the elderly population. Another option being explored is deinstitutionalization;

there are many individuals throughout the globe who perceive nursing homes should be phased out.

Phasing Out Institutionalization of the Elderly

Ageism is the stereotyping, prejudice, and discrimination toward others and oneself based on age. It is believed that more than half of the world's population is ageist against older people. In general, ageism can have the same economic, social, and psychological impacts as any other form of discrimination. With this concept in mind, several organizations and state governments have presented the concept of deinstitutionalization regarding nursing homes. Some of the supporters of this process are stating that careful planning and slow implementation of the closing of nursing homes should be the recommended strategy; to avoid the same adversities that transpired with the closing of state-funded psychiatric institutions.

A systematic review and meta-analysis was conducted in order to answer the focused question: does institutionalization interfere with the elderly's quality of life? The conclusion was that institutionalization influences negatively the quality of life for the elderly; questionnaire results revealed on "past, present, and future activities," that the "intimacy," "social participation," and "sensory abilities" domains demonstrated worse quality of life for the institutionalized elderly than for the non-institutionalized ones.[18]

US Deinstitutionalization of Nursing Homes

Expanding LTC residential home and community-based services has been being addressed for several years in response to consumer preferences to live in the least restrictive environment. Benefit options that states can implore to improve healthcare community-based services (HCBS) are the HCBS State Plan Option, the Community First Choice Option, the Money Follows the Person (MFP) Demonstration, and the State Balancing Incentive Program.[19] It is believed that gerontological care reform involves a culture change and that these options can assist in obtaining LTC services that rebalance elder care provisions.

Robert Applebaum, a professor at the Scripps Gerontology Center at Miami University in Ohio, stated,

> Over the last two decades, there's been a tremendous change in the long-term service system. Even in a state like Ohio, where the nursing homes were a really quite a powerful entity, we're now serving more older people at home or with home community-based services than we are in nursing homes.[20]

The population-adjusted supply of nursing home beds declined from 2011 to 2019 for 86.4% of US counties, by a mean (SD) of *129.9 (123.8) beds per*

US Nursing Home Beds per 1,000 People in 2022

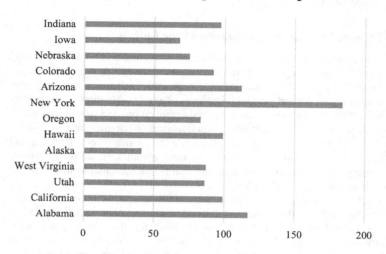

Figure 5.1 2022 Nursing Home Beds in the United States.[23]

Source: Statista. This depicts a bar graph that contains a vertical axis of specific US states and a horizontal axis of numbers 0–200, identifying the number of nursing home beds per 1,000 people, with Alaska having the lowest number below 50 beds and New York having the highest number of beds around 180.

10,000 adults aged 65 years or older per county from a baseline mean (SD) of 552.5 (274.4) beds per 10,000 adults aged 65 years or older per county in 2011.[21] In 2022, the average number of certified nursing facility beds in the United States was 106 beds per 1,000 people.[22] Figure 5.1 illustrates the number of beds in specific states per 1,000 people.

Organizations like Northeast Independent Living Services (NEILS) in Missouri support the nursing home transition/deinstitutionalization process endorsing that individuals deserve to live in the least restrictive environment, assisting people in all stages of the aging process to obtain community living and care services.

Deinstitutionalization of Nursing Homes in Other Countries

The Disability Justice Network in Ontario, Canada, is working to deinstitutionalize disabled people and the elderly stating that the current system isolates, segregates, and warehouses disabled people and elders. It is recommended that reimagining of the Canada Health Act to nationalize home care,

Number of European Care Home Beds in 2022

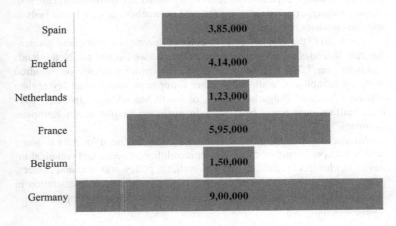

Figure 5.2 Number of Care Home Beds in European Countries in 2022.[28]

Source: Statista. This funnel diagram portrays a vertical axis of European Countries and the number of care home beds is portrayed, with Germany having the most beds at 900,000 and the Netherlands having the least at 123,000.

palliative care, pharmacare, and funding for assistive devices should be created and implemented in the country, further stating, "We believe that disabled people and elders are valuable apart from their ability to produce. We should not segregate people based on their ability to contribute to the economy."[24]

The Netherlands and Germany

A study of deinstitutionalization of nursing homes in the Netherlands and Germany revealed that in-home care is found to be less costly and enhances the dignity of life of elderly citizens. In Germany, there was an increase of 85.6% in the number of elderly individuals receiving in-home care covered by the country's LTC insurance, demonstrating an overall trend in the decrease of institutionalization regarding the gerontological population.[25] Elderly in-home care also has increased in the Netherlands by 65.6%; relatively less elderly people are spending their days in institutions.[26]

Additional European Countries

Since 2016, elder care systems have supported deinstitutionalization in Finland where nursing home care is being replaced by in-home care and creation of home-like housing units. In 2019, 70% of elder care users received care at home or in the community in OECD countries.[27] Deinstitutionalization of care and the major expansion of community-based and home-based care provisions are supported in these countries. The numbers of care home beds in specific countries are depicted in Figure 5.2.

As of 2018, the number of LTC beds in European nursing and residential care facilities varied greatly. For instance, Sweden and the Netherlands had both over 1,300 LTC beds in nursing and residential care per hundred thousand inhabitants, while some other European countries had fewer than 100 beds, such as Bulgaria, Greece, or North Macedonia.[29] In 2022, over three million care home beds were in operation in just seven European countries.[30]

An article written by WHO, discussing the growing need for elder in-home care in Europe, identified changes in epidemiology, science and technical innovation, changes in attitudes and expectations, policy priorities and choices, demographic shifts, and social changes as factors related to an alteration in elder care service provisions,[31] addressing systemic reform to improve elder quality of care.

US Funding for In-Home Care

Colorado participates in a Medicaid-funded program called MFP that provides funding for moving elderly or disabled people out of institutions and into community-based residential settings. On March 31, 2022, CMS notified current MFP grantees that it was increasing the reimbursement rate for MFP "supplemental services." These services are now 100% federally funded with no state share. CMS also announced that it was expanding the definition of supplemental services to include additional services that can support an individual's transition from an institution to the community, including short-term housing and food assistance.[32]

Also, addressing nursing home challenges, states are exploring how Medicaid options can support people with LTC needs through consumer direction programs that allow family members to be paid for providing care. States have developed and expanded consumer direction programs over the past decades; given the increased interest in home- and community-based care over institutional care, consumer direction programs are a growing option to offer older adults and people with disabilities an alternative to institutionalization. Advocates for the phasing out of nursing homes strongly present that there needs to be an increase of stay-at-home elder supports in all communities, and better-funded in-home care programs through increased revisions to American Medicare and Medicaid participation requirements that support the phasing out of nursing homes. There are other processes that can be utilized to assist in phasing out of nursing homes such as dementia units, in-home hospice services, PACE programs, and subacute units.

Additional Programs/Structures That Can Assist in the Phasing Out of Nursing Homes

Nursing homes currently have skilled units that provide care to patients post-acute, such as rehabilitation services, intravenous therapy, wound treatment, and so on. Restructuring of acute care hospitals that provide extended services on a subacute unit could phase out this service in LTC. A subacute unit in a hospital setting provides services for patients who still require treatment, but who do not require continuous in-hospital services.

Hospice Services

Another option to assist in the phasing out of nursing homes is the utilization of in-home hospice care programs; there is provision for Medicare-certified hospice care in the residential home, when qualified. There is no cost for hospice care; there is a copayment of $5 for each prescription for outpatient drugs for pain and symptom management. Items Medicare will not cover once the hospice benefit starts are treatments and prescription drugs intended to cure a person's terminal illness or care from any provider that was not set up by the hospice team.

Dementia Facilities

Memory care units/facilities are a form of residential LTC that provides intensive, specialized care for people with Alzheimer's disease or dementia. Dementia facilities are usually smaller in size housing below 20 beds and provide assistance with basic activities of daily living (ADLs), meals, housekeeping, transportation, and recreational activities. These facilities are more secure and supervised; preventing residents from getting lost. In addition, they offer structured environments and activities that reduce stress and are designed for memory loss.

Program of All Inclusive Care for the Elderly (PACE) Programs

PACE is a Medicare and Medicaid program that helps individuals meet their health care needs in the community versus going to a nursing home. It provides medical and social services to elderly individuals still living in the community, and anything else the healthcare professionals on a PACE team decide a person may need to improve and maintain their health. This includes prescription drugs and any *medically necessary* care.

In Oregon, Providence ElderPlace is a PACE Program that provides medical care, medications, medical supplies, adult day care, in-home care, care coordination, transportation, and more for qualified individuals in their populace. In addition, their adult day programs provide a supportive environment for older adults who benefit from extra care, activities, and social stimulation.

Advocates

There are many organizations that act as advocates for residents in LTC facilities. The Ombudsman is probably the most active and well-known among nursing home employees; they visit nursing homes frequently in many states. All 50 states, the District of Columbia, Guam, and Puerto Rico have an LTC ombudsman program to improve gerontological care at local and national levels. A former Indiana State Long-Term Care Ombudsman and president of the National Association of State Long-Term Care Ombudsman Programs stated:

> This is the time when we can get some real improvements in terms of staffing in the nursing homes. As you know, this has been a problem for decades and it just became absolutely exacerbated during the pandemic.[33]

The National Citizens' Coalition for Nursing Home Care Reform (NCCNHR) addresses public concerns about nursing home conditions and substandard healthcare in the United States. The coalition comprises Citizen Advocacy Groups (CAGs) who are citizens formulating processes to improve resident quality of care in nursing homes, typically the members have a family member/friend in a facility. The organization provides a toolkit to the CAGs, "Organizing to Improve Long-Term Care in Your State & Community: A NCCNHR Toolkit for Citizen Advocates" that provides guidance in four areas: basic elements, fundraising, technology, and culture change. A longtime nursing home advocate with the New Jersey office of the LTC ombudsman program and the state LTC ombudsman stated:

> I felt like we were abandoning the people in long-term care. I felt like they were being left to their own devices, and I knew it was going to be bad.[34]

California Advocates for Nursing Home Reform (CANHR) was established in 1983 to improve the choices, care, and quality of life for LTC consumers and seek humane alternatives to institutionalization. The Long-Term Care Community Coalition is based out of New York and focuses on improving quality of care, life, and dignity for residents in LTC. A member of the New York State Assembly and chair of the NYS Assembly Health Committee stated:

> Virtually every problem with COVID in our nursing homes was a problem that had been long existing in our nursing homes. COVID just made all those problems worse, and for some people made them more evident.[35]

Other Countries

In Ontario, Canada, "Concerned Friends" is an advocacy group that focuses on important issues in the LTC industry and relays their concerns to governmental officials. Care Home Advocates are utilized in the United Kingdom to assist nursing home residents in exploring options and making informed decisions, such as The Advonet Group.

In Ireland, Sage Advocacy has secured funding from the Irish Human Rights and Equality Commission under its Human Rights and Equality Grants Scheme 2021–2022 on a project called "Establishing an Observatory on Human-Rights in Long-Term Care in Ireland." One of the key objectives of this project is to give people who experience LTC and support services the opportunity to have their voices heard and affect change. This project is concentrated on recipients of LTC and support services.[36]

We have examined several solutional components encompassing the provisions of elder care that could be incorporated into gerontological provisions worldwide. A serious evaluation of the LTC industry in each specific country needs to be conducted to assist in moving forward to prepare for future public health emergencies. I do not believe that there is any one model of gerontological care that could be generically feasible for all circumstances; thus, each government needs to evaluate its current elder care provisions and establish short and long-term goals to improve medical, social, and mental health provisions in the industry for future pandemics.

Notes

1 Harrison, Stephanie, et al. (2019). Alternative staffing structures in a clustered domestic model in residential aged care in Australia. *Australasian Journal on Ageing*. 38(Suppl 2). https://doi.org/10.1111/ajag.12674. (accessed November 4, 2023). pp. 68–74.

2 The Green House Project. (2023). Green house homes and COVID: More than just a design. https://thegreenhouseproject.org/wp-content/uploads/Green-House-Homes-and-COVID-1.pdf. (accessed November 4, 2023).

3 Waters, Rob. (2021). The big idea behind a new model of small nursing homes. *Health Affairs*. 40(3). https://www.healthaffairs.org/doi/10.1377/hlthaff.2021.00081. (accessed July 3, 2023).

4 Zhu, Xuemei, et al. (2022). Nursing home design and COVID-19: Implications for guidelines and regulation. *Journal of the American Medical Directors Association*. 23(2):e1. https://pubmed.ncbi.nlm.nih.gov/34990585/. (accessed July 3, 2023), pp. 272–279.

5 Ontario Newsroom. (2022). Ontario increasing construction funding for long-term care homes. https://news.ontario.ca/en/release/1002523/ontario-increasing-construction-funding-for-long-term-care-homes. (accessed July 3, 2023).

6 Bachman, Marta, et al. (2021). The increasing investment of real estate in the health system – A comparison between the USA and Europe. *Healthcare*. 9(12). https://doi.org/10.3390/healthcare9121633. (accessed November 4, 2023). p. 1633.

7 European Commission. (2019). EIB grants 57.5 million euros under Investment Plan to Vitalia home to build 19 retirement homes in Spain.

https://ec.europa.eu/commission/presscorner/detail/en/IP_19_6835. (accessed July 3, 2023).
8 European Commission. (2019). EIB grants 57.5 million euros under Investment Plan to Vitalia home to build 19 retirement homes in Spain. https://ec.europa.eu/commission/presscorner/detail/en/IP_19_6835. (accessed July 3, 2023).
9 Royal Commission into Aged Care Quality and Safety. (2020). Capital financing for residential aged care. https://agedcare.royalcommission.gov.au/sites/default/files/2020–09/capital-financing-for-residential-aged-care_0.pdf#:~: text=In%202019%2C%20the%20Aged%20Care%20Financing%20Authority%20estimated,care%20places%20over%20the%20decade%20to%2030June%202020. (accessed July 3, 2023).
10 Royal Commission into Aged Care Quality and Safety. (2020). Capital financing for residential aged care. https://agedcare.royalcommission.gov.au/sites/default/files/2020-09/capital-financing-for-residential-aged-care_0.pdf#:~: text=In%202019%2C%20the%20Aged%20Care%20Financing%20Authority%20estimated,care%20places%20over%20the%20decade%20to%2030June%202020. (accessed July 3, 2023).
11 Gill, Dee. (2021). Codifying the nursing home industry's elusive, alarming turnover rates, Payroll data allows researchers to finally build an accurate and meaningful measurement. https://anderson-review.ucla.edu/codifying-the-nursing-home-industrys-elusive-alarming-turnover-rates/. (accessed November 4, 2023).
12 Jividen, Sarah R. N. (2021). CNA turnover costs: Pain points for skilled nursing facilities. https://www.relias.com/blog/cna-turnover-costs-for-skilled-nursing-facilities#:~:text=Significant%20pain%20points%20of%20CNA%20turnover%20costs%20include,solutions%20include%20CNA%20empowerment%20and%20preventing%20clinician%20burnout. (accessed July 7, 2023).
13 Anderson-Mutch, Kimberly. (2022). How to reduce staff turn-over in skilled nursing facilities. *SmartLinx.* www.smartlinx.com/resources/blog/how-to-reduce-staff-turnover-in-skilled-nurse-facilities. (accessed July 7, 2023).
14 Castle, N. G. (2001). Administrator turnover and quality of care in nursing homes. *Gerontologis.* 41(6). https://pubmed.ncbi.nlm.gov/11723344/. (accessed July 7, 2023). pp. 757–767.
15 Miller, Joel. (2022). *How to Improve Mental Health and Substance Use Care for Older Adults.* National Council on Aging. https://ncoa.org/article/how-to-improve-access-to-mental-health-and-substance-use-care-for-older-adults. (accessed July 7, 2023).
16 The Canadian Academy of Geriatric Psychiatry (CAGP) and Canadian Coalition for Seniors Mental Health (CCMSH). (2021). Mental health care in long-term care during COVID-19 position paper. https://ccsmh.ca/wp-content/uploads/2021/01/COVID-19-Mental-Health-in-LTC-Web.pdf. (accessed November 5, 2023).
17 United Nations. (2020). Policy brief: COVID-19 and the need for action on mental health. https://unsdg.un.org/resources/policy-brief-covid-19-and-need-action-mental-health. (accessed July 7, 2023).

18 de Medeiros, Mariana Marinho Davino, et al. (2020). Does the in-stitutionalization influence elderly's quality of life? A systematic review and meta – analysis. *BMC Geriatrics.* 20. https://doi.org/10.1186/s12877-020-1452-0. (accessed July 8, 2023). p. 44.
19 The Commonwealth Fund. (2023). National health reform and long-term care. www.commonwealthfund.org/publications/newsletter-article/national-health-reform-and-long-term-care. (accessed December 26, 2023).
20 Schulson, Michael. (2020). Coronavirus is renewing a call to abolish nursing homes. *Quartz.* https://qz.com/1872956/is-there-a-better-alternative-to-nursing-homes. (accessed July 8, 2023).
21 Miller, Katherine, E. M., et al. (2023). Trends in supply of nurs-ing home beds, 2011–2019. *JAMA Network Open.* 1;6(3):e230640. www.ncbi.nlm.nih.gov/pmc/articles/PMC9978943/#:~:text=The%20population-adjusted%20supply%20of%20nursing%20home%20beds%20declined,65%20years%20or%20older%20per%20county%20in%202011. (accessed July 8, 2023).
22 Statista. (2022). Average number of certified nursing facility beds in the United States in 2022, per state. www.statista.com/statistics/323253/average-number-of-certified-nursing-facility-beds-in-the-united-states-by-state/. (accessed July 8, 2023).
23 Statista. (2022). Average number of certified nursing facility beds in the United States in 2022, per state. www.statista.com/statistics/323253/average-number-of-certified-nursing-facility-beds-in-the-united-states-by-state/. (accessed July 8, 2023).
24 Disability Justice Network of Ontario. (2023). Demanding decarceration of long-term care. www.djno.ca/decarceration-of-ltc. (accessed July 8, 2023).
25 Loman, R. M. J. (2019). Deinstitutionalization of long-term care for older adults: A comparison study between Germany and the Netherlands. https://essay.utwente.nl/80257/1/Loman_MA_EuropeanStudies.pdf. (accessed July 8, 2023). pp. 41–45.
26 Loman, RMJ. (2019). Deinstitutionalization of long-term care for older adults: A comparison study between Germany and the Netherlands. https://essay.utwente.nl/80257/1/Loman_MA_EuropeanStudies.pdf. (accessed July 8, 2023). pp. 41–45.
27 Glinskaya, Elena. (2019). Government stewardship of elderly care. *Worldbank.* https://hedocs.worldbank.org/en/doc/650961574287997386-0160022019/original/SPJCC19PCCD3S3GlinskayaGovernmentStew-ardshipofElderlyCare.pdf. (accessed July 8, 2023).
28 Statista. (2022). Countries with the most care home beds in Europe in 2022. www.statista.com/statistics/1366427/countries-with-the-most-care-home-beds-in-europe/#:~:text=In%202022%2C%20over%20three%20million%20care%20home%20beds,home%20beds%2C%20with%20595%-20thousand%20beds%20in%202022. (accessed July 8, 2023).
29 Statista. (2021). Residential care in Europe – statistics & facts. www.statista.com/topics/7965/residential-care-in-europe/#topicOverview. (accessed July 8, 2023).
30 Statista. (2022). Countries with the most care home beds in Europe in 2022. www.statista.com/statistics/1366427/countries-with-the-most-care-

home-beds-in-europe/#:~:text=In%202022%2C%20over%20three%20
million%20care%20home%20beds,home%20beds%2C%20with%20
595%20thousand%20beds%20in%202022. (accessed July 8, 2023).

31 Tarricone, Rosanna, and Tsouros, Agis. (2008). Home care in Europe: The
    solid facts. World Health Organization, Regional Office for Europe. https://
    apps.who.int/iris/handle/10665/328766. (accessed July 12, 2022), p. 3.

32 Medicaid. (2022). Money follows the person. https://www.medicaid.
    gov/medicaid/long-term-services-supports/money-follows-person/index.
    html. (accessed July 8, 2023).

33 Nursing Home 411. (2022). I feel like I'm in a prison: An oral history
    of COVID-19 in nursing homes. Long Term Care Community Coalition
    Interviews. www.nursinghome411.org/oral-history/. (retrieved July 12,
    2022).

34 Nursing Home 411. (2022). I feel like I'm in a prison: An oral history
    of COVID-19 in nursing homes. Long Term Care Community Coalition
    Interviews. www.nursinghome411.org/oral-history/. (retrieved July 12,
    2022).

35 Nursing Home 411. (2022). I feel like I'm in a prison: An oral history
    of COVID-19 in nursing homes. Long Term Care Community Coalition
    Interviews. www.nursinghome411.org/oral-history/. (retrieved July 12,
    2022).

36 Sage Advocacy. (2022). An introduction to the project: Establishing an
    observatory on human rights in long-term care. www.sageadvocacy.ie/re-
    sources/establishing-an-observatory-on-human-rights-in-long-term-care.
    (accessed November 27, 2022).

6 Organizations Globally
Preparing for Future Pandemics

The COVID-19 pandemic brought about many ongoing challenges worldwide. IPC organizations and many other institutions throughout the globe have formulated strategies on ways to improve transmission prevention, surveillance, pandemic preparedness, international collaboration, workforce challenges, public health communication, universal health coverage, manufacturing, and a much-needed increased focus on low- and middle-income countries for future public health emergencies. The strategies that have been or will be implemented by the CDC, WHO, PPF, and ECDC impact the healthcare industry as a whole and the LTC industry for future pandemics.

The Center for Global Development hosted an event in July 2023, titled, *What's Next? The Frequency and Scale of Future Pandemics*, elaborating on information that a team at Metabiota (a biotechnology company in San Francisco, California, that compiles data from around the world to predict disease outbreaks) presented predicting that the next pandemic might not be as far away as we think, they estimate that the probability of a future zoonotic spillover event resulting in a pandemic of COVID-19 magnitude or larger is between 2.5% and 3.3% annually; in other words, there is a 22–28% chance that another outbreak on the magnitude of COVID-19 will occur within the next ten years, and a 47–57% chance it will occur within the next 25 years.[1] The ECDC acknowledges that pandemics will occur in the future and has established additional protocols for PHE preparation.

European Centre for Disease Prevention and Control

ECDC explains that preparing for a pandemic is a continuous process of planning, exercising, revising, and translating into action national and subnational pandemic preparedness and response plans, describing that key elements of a pandemic preparedness cycle include strategic planning, operational planning, exercises and reviews, implementation, and evaluation.[2] And, it also further elaborates that pandemic preparedness is most effective if it is built on general principles that guide preparedness planning for any acute threat to public health.[3]

DOI: 10.4324/9781003466192-9

ECDC is committed to ensuring that the EU and its Member States are prepared for and enabled to respond effectively to infectious disease outbreaks and pandemics. The organization ensures that preventative actions are taken in advance of outbreaks, which include:

1. Providing assessments of preparedness capacities in EU/EEA Member States
2. Identification and sharing of good practices, such as evidence-based tools and guidance, especially for national emergency planning
3. Identifying, prioritizing, and understanding risks and vulnerabilities
4. Developing and appraising the evidence base surrounding the effectiveness of infectious disease control and PHSM
5. Assisting in preparedness of workforce capacity building through training and the development of training curricula[4]

COVID-19 Assessment

As part of the efforts to further strengthen future pandemic preparedness, ECDC visited six EU/EEA countries between June and September 2022: Austria, Estonia, Finland, Greece, Latvia, and Romania. These Member States accepted the ECDC initiative and responded positively to the proposed visit by experts from the Agency, to facilitate high-level discussions on lessons learned from the COVID-19 pandemic, including international coordination and recommendations for future ECDC support.

The lessons learned from the COVID-19 pandemic included: the need for updated, generic/all-hazard, flexible, scalable preparedness plans; the need for an addition of formalized roles of public health in decision-making and crisis management structures; the necessity to stress the importance of intersectoral work in the preparedness and response to public health crises; the need to organize procedures to achieve surge capacity for staff (HCWs, public health staff) ahead of a crisis; a necessity that during preparedness planning to update legislation governing communicable disease control, taking into account ethics/human rights, intersectoral effects, and the outlining of responsibilities including international cooperation; and the need for improvement in coordination and solidarity.[5] The following actions are the results from these visits:

- Develop guidance on generic preparedness planning, based on the lessons identified.
- Facilitate the sharing of national preparedness plans among the Member States.
- Facilitate intersectoral advice and work with stakeholders and experts outside the public health sector.
- Organize a feedback mechanism for ECDC outputs.
- Provide assistance to conduct simulation exercises by offering staff training or training material.

- Continue work with countries to perform in-action reviews and after-action reviews, as requested.
- Facilitate evaluation and monitoring of the implementation of nonpharmaceutical interventions (NPIs) (e.g., development of guidance and/or training).
- Define indicators for preparedness planning.

And, assess all the Member States' prevention, preparedness, and response plans every three years.[6]

Improved Surveillance

In the EU, there was also the creation of the European Commission's Directorate General European Health Emergency Preparedness and Response Authority (HERA), the European Health Union, and the regulation on serious cross-border threats to health came into force.[7]

Surveillance was identified as an area needing improvement during the COVID-19 pandemic.

Secure and interoperable digital platforms and applications in support of epidemiological surveillance are crucial at the EU level. ECDC has the task of developing such systems, and it will seek solutions that allow better use of the data by applying new digital technologies, such as artificial intelligence and computer modeling in data compilation and analysis.[8] Improving epidemiological surveillance through the digitalization of integrated surveillance systems in the EU countries will constitute the basis for an EU-level digitalized surveillance system of communicable diseases, with interoperability across borders.[9]

Interconnected systems would ease monitoring of the impact of communicable disease crises (e.g., pandemics) on the healthcare system/hospitals in the future. The enhanced capacity to obtain a comprehensive overview of the epidemiological situation at the EU level, to monitor the impact of communicable disease events on the healthcare system, and the possibility to anticipate future trends should be the EU-added value of surveillance of which the outcomes will be made available to decision-makers at EU and national levels.[10]

ECDC further elaborates that international cooperation and solidarity among countries are also important, and reportedly, in many cases, this was not optimal during the COVID-19 pandemic. International cooperation needs to be improved during peacetime, and agreements need to be developed and implemented for the sharing of data, equipment, and even resources.

Centers for Disease Control and Prevention

Addressing the US House of Representatives Subcommittee on Health—Committee on Energy and Commerce in May 2023, the CDC presented that the team was working hard to address the challenges identified during the COVID-19 pandemic. And, that they were building on a strong foundation of core capabilities in public health and leveraging their areas of expertise and successes to build systems that are more resilient and can better respond and adapt to emergencies. The CDC also stated to the House of Representatives that while the COVID-19 pandemic was the most serious public health event in over 100 years, the increased frequency of infectious disease outbreaks should highlight the sobering reality that we should not be asking if we will face another serious public health threat, but when,[11] further elaborating on areas of focus for improvement including improved laboratory services, healthcare workforce improvements, upgraded integrated data platforms, enhanced international cooperation, enhancing elements identified off of internal reviews, and implementation of the Center for Forecasting and Outbreak Analytics (CFA).

Improved Laboratory Services

Beginning with COVID-19, the Sequencing for Public Health Emergency Response, Epidemiology, and Surveillance consortium engaged academic and private sector sequencing laboratories to help the CDC monitor changes in the virus, gain important insights to support contact tracing efforts, provide crucial information to aid in identifying diagnostic and therapeutic targets, and advance public health research in the areas about transmission dynamics, host response, and evolution of the virus. The Centers of Excellence will extend these partnerships and help CDC leverage state-of-the-art laboratory technology and public health innovation to continue to advance genomic surveillance.[12]

Healthcare Workforce Improvements

The CDC recognizes the healthcare workforce challenges and has made substantial one-time investments to address these long-standing needs, including $2 billion for immediate emergency crisis response and $3 billion in foundational workforce and infrastructure. These funds not only provide critical support for school-based health programs, public health professional development, and acquisition of important technological upgrades but also allow state and local jurisdictions to build their workforce to best serve their communities.[13]

Upgraded Integrated Data Platforms

The Response Ready Enterprise Data Integration (RREDI) platform, which is the next generation of HHS Protect, is a secure decision-making and operations platform developed for the whole-of-government response to the COVID-19 pandemic. RREDI uses and integrates data from more than

300 sources across federal, state, and local governments and the healthcare industry and is accessible to 4,500+ unique users across 30+ federal agencies, 56 states and territories, and the private sector.[14]

In addition, CDC's NHSN has provided essential data on known and emerging threats from more than 38,000 American healthcare facilities, including the US government's first comprehensive look at pathogen-agnostic hospital bed occupancy and capacity data from all US hospitals. CDC continues to leverage systems like NHSN to meet the goals of the National Biodefense Strategy and to build on the lessons learned from the COVID-19 pandemic to maintain and enhance an enduring domestic all-hazards hospital data collection capability.[15]

International Cooperation

In the fight against infectious diseases, no nation can stand alone. When it takes less than 36 hours for an outbreak to spread from a remote village to any major city in the world, protecting US health and national security means making sure that other countries have the knowledge and the resources to stop threats before they can spread beyond their borders. Together, we must build these first lines of defense to better prevent, detect, and respond to disease and other biothreats.[16]

Internal Review

The future CDC must be prepared to lead the country in core capabilities and to set themselves up for success. In the spring of 2022, a launched extensive review of the agency's organizational structures, systems, and processes to strengthen its ability to deliver on its core mission to equitably protect the health, safety, and security of Americans began. In August 2022, based on this review and other substantial internal and external input, a CDC Moving Forward initiative was launched that focused on the following top improvement areas, as illustrated in Figure 6.1.

Center for CFA

In April 2022, the Center for CFA was created to improve the nation's ability to prepare for and respond to infectious disease threats using data, modeling, and analytics, due to the course of the COVID-19 pandemic in the United States being hampered by data-collection problems. The goal of the **Center for CFA** is to enable timely, effective decision-making to improve outbreak response using data, modeling, and analytics. To do so, CFA produces models and forecasts to characterize the state of an outbreak and its course, inform public health decision-makers on the potential consequences of deploying

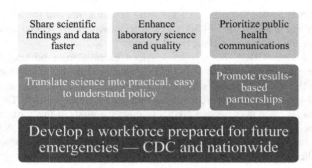

Figure 6.1 CDC Improvement Strategies for Future Pandemics.[17]

Source: Centers for Disease Control and Prevention. This design art contains six boxes formatted in a rectangle that display CDC improvements for future pandemics.

control measures, and support innovation to continuously improve the science of outbreak analytics and modeling.[18]

World Health Organization

In May 2022, WHO launched the first-ever global IPC report. Dr. Tedros Adhanom Ghebreyesus, WHO Director General, stated, "The COVID-19 pandemic has exposed many challenges and gaps in IPC in all regions and countries, including those which had the most advanced IPC programs."[19] The report revealed that high-income countries were more likely to be progressing their IPC work, and are eight times more likely to have a more advanced IPC implementation status than low-income countries, leading to the development of the Preparedness and Resilience for Emerging Threats (PRET) Initiative.

Preparedness and Resilience for Emerging Threats

In April 2023, WHO launched the PRET Initiative; PRET is an evolution in WHO's approach to pandemic preparedness through the application of a mode of transmission lens. A Call to Action entailing a collective commitment on specific actions to obtain progress by December 2025 with regard to pandemics included the following:

1. Update preparedness plans that affirm priority actions.
2. Increase connectivity among stakeholders in pandemic preparedness planning through systematic coordination and cooperation.
3. Dedicate sustained investments, financing, and monitoring of pandemic preparedness.[20]

PRET builds on the current momentum to strengthen the global architecture for health security and operationalizes the vision of a more equitable and robust response to future disease pandemics. Drawing upon lessons from previous events and identified gaps and opportunities, PRET helps stakeholders to converge resources and ensure that there are:

- Clarity on implementation priorities as established by country authorities and in line with regional and global mandates
- Increased opportunity for collaboration
- Common and systematic roll-out of resources that facilitates cross-country and cross-stakeholder actions.[21]

WHO is the specialized health agency of the United Nations.

The United Nations

In September 2023, the first-ever head-of-state summit on pandemic prevention, preparedness, and response was held at the United Nations General Assembly to strengthen international cooperation, coordination, governance, and investment needed to prevent a repeat of the devastating health, and socioeconomic impacts caused by COVID-19, approving a political declaration. The declaration addressed numerous issues, including:

1. Protect our communities through investing in primary healthcare and other health system measures, as part of a commitment to universal health coverage, so as to ensure that robust national health systems are in place to respond to future pandemics.
2. Invest in ensuring that WHO is strengthened to the level needed to play its role in responding to pandemic threats. Sustainable financing of WHO, and national health systems, is essential for making the world safer.
3. Strengthen health workforce and rapid response capacities, surveillance and supply systems, and local manufacturing abilities, to enable and empower all countries to have the ability to meet their own needs to prevent, prepare for, and respond to pandemics.
4. Scale up health system capacities to address pandemic threats in low- and lower-middle-income countries, especially across Africa.
5. Counter and address the negative impacts of health-related misinformation, disinformation, hate speech, and stigmatization, especially on social media platforms, on people's physical and mental health, in order to strengthen pandemic prevention, preparedness, and response and foster trust in public health systems and authorities.
6. Leverage the potential of the multilateral system and scale up the multisectoral approach needed to improve pandemic prevention, preparedness, and response, due to the multifaceted causes and consequences of

pandemics, which support the attainment of the Sustainable Development Goals.[22]

The Global Preparedness Monitoring Board (GPMB) is an independent monitoring and accountability body co-convened by the World Bank and the WHO.

Global Preparedness Monitoring Board

GPMB's 2020 report, *A World in Disorder*, notes how the COVID-19 pandemic revealed a collective failure to take pandemic prevention, preparedness, and response seriously and prioritize it accordingly. The 2023 publication, *Preventing, Preparing, and Responding (PPR) to Disease Outbreaks and Pandemics: Future Directions for World Bank Group*, outlines an agenda to support PPR enhancement at country, regional, and global levels as part of a broader approach to strengthen health systems through actions in three interconnected domains: financing; global engagements and partnership; and analytics, evidence, and dialogue.[23]

Also, in *Putting Pandemics Behind Us: Investing in One Health to Reduce Risks of Emerging Infectious Diseases*, policymakers, governments, and the international community are urged to invest in pandemic prevention and to move away from the business-as-usual approach based on containment and control after a disease has emerged. The report estimates that prevention costs guided by a One Health approach—which would sustainably balance and optimize the health of people, animals, and ecosystems—would range from $10.3 billion to $11.5 billion per year, compared with the cost of managing pandemics which, according to the recent estimate by the G20 Joint Finance and Health Taskforce, amounts to about $30.1 billion per year.[24]

"Prevention is better than cure. COVID-19 has shown that a pandemic risk anywhere becomes a pandemic risk everywhere. The economic case for One Health is powerful—the cost of prevention is extremely modest compared to the cost of managing and responding to pandemics," said Mari Pangestu, World Bank Managing Director of Development Policy and Partnerships.[25]

The One Health approach is a collaborative approach for strengthening systems to prevent, prepare, and respond to infectious diseases and related issues such as antimicrobial resistance that threatens human, animal, and environmental health and recognizing that animal, human, and planetary health are interconnected. The report, *Putting Pandemics Behind Us: Investing in One Health to Reduce Risks of Emerging Infectious Diseases*, highlights that investing in One Health is an investment in humanity's future; it is holistic and assists governments, international organizations, and donors to direct financial resources to optimize scarce funding resources and prevent pandemics.

Pan American Health Organization (PAHO)

PAHO is the specialized health agency of the International American System and also serves as the regional office for the Americas of WHO, which engages in technical cooperation with its member countries to fight communicable diseases and noncommunicable diseases and their causes, to strengthen health systems, and to respond to emergencies and disasters.

In Washington, DC, on May 12, 2023, PAHO revealed that between 600,000 and 2 million more healthcare professionals, including nurses, are needed to meet the health needs of the population of the Americas. The nursing situation in the Americas is illustrated in Figure 6.2.

> A well-educated, skilled, and equitably distributed workforce is critical to building resilient health systems, meeting population health needs, and better preparing for future threats and pandemics.
>
> PAHO Director, Dr. Jarbas Barbosa[27]

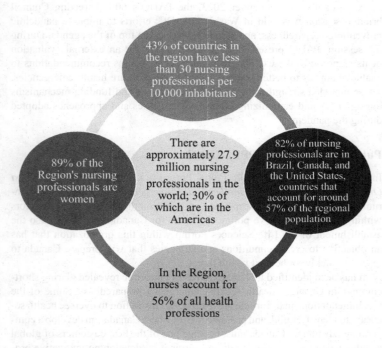

Figure 6.2 Nursing Situation in the Americas.[26]

Source: Pan American Health Organization. This image/design art contains a circular depiction of five round or oval sections that illustrate the current America's nursing status and shortage.

In Brasilia, Brazil, on July 3, 2023, the Director of the PAHO, Dr. Jarbas Barbosa, took part in the 17th National Health Conference; the event is one of the country's most important on public health. During the Conference, the PAHO director highlighted that now that COVID-19 has left its acute phase, it is essential that all lessons learned are transformed into actions so that the world is better prepared for future emergencies that may arise; Dr. Barbosa stated:

> This is the least we can do to honor the millions of people who died during the pandemic, as well as the health workers who did not shy away from providing care, even while risking their own lives.[28]

Dr. Barbosa also highlighted the need for Latin America and the Caribbean to produce more vaccines, medicines, and personal protective equipment for their populations; "poor countries had tremendous difficulty getting access."[29]

Additionally, in September 2023, the PAHO's 60th Directing Council briefing session was held in Washington, DC; efforts to improve pandemic prevention, preparedness, and response were at the top of the agenda. During the session, PAHO presented its follow-up plan for an external evaluation of its response to the COVID-19 pandemic, as well as recommendations to enable countries to better prepare and respond to future health emergencies. These included strengthening PAHO's governance and funding mechanisms during crises and capitalizing on new technologies and approaches adopted during the pandemic.[30]

Public Policy Forum (PPF) Canada

In September 2023, the Public Policy Forum in Canada released, *The Next One: Preparing Canada for another health emergency.* The Public Policy Forum is a non-partisan, member-based organization that works with all sectors within Canada to improve policy outcomes for Canadians; there is also the establishment of the Life Sciences Forum within this organization that has an objective to create conditions and strategies that will prepare Canada to respond quickly to the next health threat.

It has been identified that the COVID-19 pandemic revealed glaring shortcomings in Canada's health security emergency preparedness. Some of the recommendations in the article are to create an institution to oversee health security; to identify, build, and promote niches where Canada can develop a comparative advantage; Canada must become one of the best customers of global supply chains for essential goods and services by developing innovative procurement mechanisms and institutionalizing those developed during the pandemic; to create standardized, anonymized electronic intelligence-gathering systems to collect and aggregate real-time data required for health emergency response decision making; to improve health emergency risk communications, integrating strategies to respond to misinformation and disinformation; and to conduct regular system readiness testing through simulations and scenarios to probe for weaknesses in preparedness.[31]

UK Health Security Agency

The UKHSA was formulated in 2021, with a central objective to help the United Kingdom prepare for future pandemics. A report submitted in March 2023, to the Science and Technology Committee, *How Prepared is the UK for the Next Pandemic?*, revealed that the National Security Risk Assessment was updated to include a broader range of pathogens; the pandemic preparedness governess and assurance processes were revised; UKHSA established the Vaccine Development and Evaluation Centre (VDEC); and systems for improved surveillance, laboratory capacity, diagnostics, and technology/data were adjusted based on lessons learned from the COVID-19 pandemic. Additionally, the United Kingdom agreed to a ten-year partnership with Moderna, which will invest in mRNA research and development in the United Kingdom. In addition, the Training and Exercising team within the UKHSA Emergency, Preparedness, Resilience, and Response Directorate (ESPRR) will regularly test and be exercised to test for infectious disease response preparedness.[32]

The first report from the United Kingdom on the G7 (Group of 7 is an informal grouping of seven countries: Canada, France, Germany, Italy, Japan, the United Kingdom, and the United States, as well as the EU) 100-day mission (100DM) was released in 2021, after UK Prime Minister, Boris Johnson, challenged G7 leaders to explore how to harness the unprecedented scientific innovation and public and private collaboration seen in the COVID-19 crisis to reduce the time from discovery to deployment of diagnostics, therapeutics, and vaccines (DTVs) in future health crises to 100 days, thus assisting with reducing the impact of future pandemics.[33] The United Kingdom, as G7 President, has worked with G7 leaders, the WHO, and global 100DM implementing partners to mobilize delivery through a systematic approach to implementation, across three lines of engagement:

1. Broadening international political, institutional, and scientific support for the Mission and its recommendations
2. Convening and mobilizing organizations responsible for leading the implementation of the specific 100DM recommendations
3. Calling on G7 Governments to take concrete action domestically to bolster support for the 100DM[34]

In March 2022, the Coalition for Epidemic Preparedness Innovations (CEPI, a global partnership launched in Davos, Switzerland, for vaccine development) and the United Kingdom cohosted the Global Pandemic

Preparedness Summit in London, United Kingdom. Issues addressed at the summit were the 100DM, improving equitable access, boosting vaccine manufacturing, and the fact that global pandemic preparedness needs global collaboration. The world's continued vulnerability to health, economic, and social impacts from pandemics was a central theme at the summit.[35]

As discussed in this chapter, multiple organizations throughout the world have evaluated and identified adversities experienced during the COVID-19 pandemic and have implemented strategies to improve responses to the next PHE in many diverse ways. In the subsequent chapters, we will explore governmental strategies to assist these organizations, countries, and communities to improve mitigation strategies for future pandemics.

Notes

1 Center for Global Development. (2023). What's next? Predicting the frequency and scale of future pandemics. https://www.cgdev.org/event/whats-next-predicting-frequency-and-scale-future-pandemics. (accessed October 8, 2023).

2 European Centre for Disease Prevention and Control. (2023). Why is pandemic preparedness planning important? https://www.ecdc.europa.eu/en/seasonal-influenza/preparedness/why-pandemic-preparedness. (accessed October 7, 2023).

3 European Centre for Disease Prevention and Control. (2023). Why is pandemic preparedness planning important?. https://www.ecdc.europa.eu/en/seasonal-influenza/preparedness/why-pandemic-preparedness. (accessed October 7, 2023).

4 European Centre for Disease Control and Prevention. (2023). What we do. www.ecdc.europa.eu/en/about-ecdc/what-we-do. (accessed July 4, 2023).

5 European Centre for Disease Prevention and Control. (2023). *Lessons from the COVID-19 Pandemic*. Stockholm: ECDC. www.ecdc.europa.eu/sites/default/files/documents/COVID-19-lessons-learned-may-2023.pdf. (accessed July 4, 2023), pp. 4, 9.

6 European Centre for Disease Prevention and Control. (2023). *Lessons from the COVID-19 Pandemic*. Stockholm: ECDC. www.ecdc.europa.eu/sites/default/files/documents/COVID-19-lessons-learned-may-2023.pdf. (accessed July 4, 2023). pp. 4, 9.

7 Kokki, Maarit, and Ammon, Andrea. (2023). Preparing Europe for future health threats and crisis-key elements of the European Centre for Disease Prevention and Control's reinforced mandate. *Eurosurveillance*. 28(3). www.ncbi.nlm.nih.gov/pmc/articles/PMC9853949/. (accessed October 7, 2023).

8 Kokki, Maarit, and Ammon, Andrea. (2023). Preparing Europe for future health threats and crisis-key elements of the European Centre for Disease Prevention and Control's reinforced mandate. *Eurosurveillance*. 28(3). www.ncbi.nlm.nih.gov/pmc/articles/PMC9853949/. (accessed October 7, 2023).

9 Kokki, Maarit, and Ammon, Andrea. (2023). Preparing Europe for future health threats and crisis-key elements of the European Centre for Disease

Prevention and Control's reinforced mandate. *Eurosurveillance*. 28(3). www.ncbi.nlm.nih.gov/pmc/articles/PMC9853949/. (accessed October 7, 2023).

10 Kokki, Maarit, and Ammon, Andrea. (2023). Preparing Europe for future health threats and crisis-key elements of the European Centre for Disease Prevention and Control's reinforced mandate. *Eurosurveillance*. 28(3). www. ncbi.nlm.nih.gov/pmc/articles/PMC9853949/. (accessed October 7, 2023).

11 Centers for Disease Control and Prevention, Washington. (2023). Preparing for and responding to future health security threats. www.cdc.gov/ washington/testimony/2023/t20230511.htm. (accessed October 7, 2023).

12 Centers for Disease Control and Prevention, Washington. (2023). Preparing for and responding to future health security threats. www.cdc.gov/ washington/testimony/2023/t20230511.htm. (accessed October 7, 2023).

13 Centers for Disease Control and Prevention, Washington. (2023). Preparing For and Responding to Future Health Security Threats. www.cdc.gov/ washington/testimony/2023/t20230511.htm. (accessed October 7, 2023).

14 Centers for Disease Control and Prevention, Washington. (2023). Preparing for and responding to future health security threats. www.cdc.gov/ washington/testimony/2023/t20230511.htm. (accessed October 7, 2023).

15 Centers for Disease Control and Prevention, Washington. (2023). Preparing for and responding to future health security threats. www.cdc.gov/ washington/testimony/2023/t20230511.htm. (accessed October 7, 2023).

16 Centers for Disease Control and Prevention, Washington. (2023). Preparing For and responding to future health security threats. www.cdc.gov/ washington/testimony/2023/t20230511.htm. (accessed October 7, 2023).

17 Centers for Disease Control and Prevention, Washington. (2023). Preparing for and responding to future health security threats. www.cdc.gov/ washington/testimony/2023/t20230511.htm. (accessed October 7, 2023).

18 Centers for Disease Control and Prevention. (2023). History of CFA. www.cdc.gov/forecast-outbreak-analytics/about/history.html. (accessed October 7, 2023).

19 World Health Organization. (2022). WHO launches first ever global report on infection prevention and control. https://www.who.int/news/ item/06-05-2022-who-launches-first-ever-global-report-on-infection-prevention-and-control. (accessed October 7, 2023).

20 World Health Organization. (2023). WHO launches new initiative to improve pandemic preparedness. www.who.int/news/item/26-04-2023-who-launches-new-initiative-to-improve-pandemic-preparedness. (accessed October 7, 2023).

21 World Health Organization. (2023). Preparedness and resilience for emerging threats (PRET). www.who.int/initiatives/preparedness-and-resilience-for-emerging-threats. (accessed October 7, 2023).

22 World Health Organization. (2023). WHO welcomes historic commitment by world leaders for greater collaboration, governance and investment to prevent, prepare for and respond to future pandemics. www.who.int/ news/item/20-09-023-who-welcomes-historic-commitment-by-world-leaders-for-greater-collaboration–governance-and-investment- to-prevent – prepare-for-and-respond-to-future-pandemics. (accessed October 7, 2023).

23 World Bank Group. (2023). Publication: Preventing, preparing, and responding (PPR) to disease outbreaks and pandemics: Future directions for World Bank Group. https://openknowledge.worldbank.org/entities/publication/4498810a-0eab-515d-ae9b-324ae9373315. (accessed October 8, 2023).

24 The World Bank. (2022). Prevent rather than fight the next pandemic with a one health approach. www.worldbank.org/en/news/press-release/2022/10/24/prevent-rather-than-fight-the-next-pandemic-with-a-one-health-approach-world-bank. (accessed October 8, 2023).

25 The World Bank. (2022). Prevent rather than fight the next pandemic with a one health approach. www.worldbank.org/en/news/press-release/2022/10/24/prevent-rather-than-fight-the-next-pandemic-with-a-one-health-approach-world-bank. (accessed October 8, 2023).

26 Pan American Health Organization. (2023). Reducing shortage of nurses key to better respond to the next pandemic. www.paho.org/en/news/12-5-2023-reducing-shortage-nurses-key-better-respond-next-pandemic. (accessed October 8, 2023).

27 Pan American Health Organization. (2023). Reducing shortage of nurses key to better respond to the next pandemic. www.paho.org/en/news/12-5-2023-reducing-shortage-nurses-key-better-respond-next-pandemic. (accessed October 8, 2023).

28 Pan American Health Organization. (2023). Lessons learned from the pandemic must be transformed into action to prepare for future health emergencies, highlights PAHO director at opening of 17th National Health Conference, in Brazil. www.paho.org/en/news/3-7-2023-lessons-pandemic-must-be-transformed-actions-prepare-future-health-emergencies. (accessed October 8, 2023).

29 Pan American Health Organization. (2023). Lessons learned from the pandemic must be transformed into action to prepare for future health emergencies, highlights PAHO director at opening of 17th National Health Conference, in Brazil. www.paho.org/en/news/3-7-2023-lessons-pandemic-must-be-transformed-actions-prepare-future-health-emergencies. (accessed October 8, 2023).

30 Pan American Health Organization. (2023). Charting a resilient future: Learning from COVID-19 for a safer tomorrow. www.paho.org/en/news/25-9-2023-charting-resilient-future-learning-covid-19-safer-tomorrow. (accessed October 8, 2023).

31 Public Policy Forum. (2023). The next one: Preparing Canada for another health emergency. https://ppforum.ca/publications/canadians-health-security/. (accessed October 8, 2023).

32 Department of Health and Social Care. (2023). How prepared is the UK for the next pandemic? https://committees.parliament.uk/writtenevidence/120589/pdf/. (accessed October 9, 2023).

33 G 7 United Kingdom. (2021). 100 day mission. https://assets.publishing.service.gov.uk/media/60c20a14e90e07438ee5748f/100_Days_Mission_to_respond_to_future_pandemic_threats__3_.pdf. (accessed October 9, 2023).

34 G 7 United Kingdom. (2021). 100 day mission. https://assets.publishing. service.gov.uk/media/60c20a14e90e07438ee5748f/100_Days_Mission_ to_respond_to_future_pandemic_threats__3_.pdf. (accessed October 9, 2023).
35 Centers for Disease Control and Prevention. (2023). The 100 days mission-2022 global pandemic preparedness summit. 29(3). https://wwwnc. cdc.gov/eid/article/29/3/22-1142_article. (accessed October 9, 2023).

Section III

Governmental Strategies for Long-Term Care Industry Reform

7   Regulatory Systems and Changes in Protocols to Prepare for Future Pandemics

Almost all countries have some type of regulating system setup that provides direction and monitoring of nursing homes and residential care homes. These entities either give direction for or conduct survey/inspection processes in elder care facilities to ensure compliance of regulatory guidelines. The systems are incorporated to maintain the health, safety, and welfare of clients who reside in nursing homes. In this chapter, we examine regulatory systems in the United States, Canada, Scotland, the United Kingdom, Italy, Germany, France, and Spain and what new regulatory protocols or systems have been implemented and/or revised to improve quality of care related to adversities identified during the COVID-19 pandemic, enhancing knowledge and preparedness for future pandemics.

The United States—HHS

In the United States, amendments to social security insurance in 1950 enabled direct payments to healthcare providers, increasing the federal government's involvement in nursing homes. The Department of HHS regulates nursing homes in America. Currently, there are over 15,000 LTC facilities in the United States that are inspected annually; each facility must have at least a standard survey (typically takes four days to complete) and a life safety code survey performed and be in compliance with requirements to receive payments under the Medicare and Medicaid programs. Deficiencies are categorized based on scope and severity as illustrated in Figure 7.1. A 2019 report that evaluated trends in deficiencies revealed:

1. The number of surveys and deficiencies increased from 2015 to 2016 and then decreased in 2017.
2. 94% of deficiencies had less serious ratings and 6% more serious ratings.
3. 31% of nursing homes had a deficiency type cited at least five times during the review period.
4. Ten states accounted for half of the deficiencies identified.[1]

DOI: 10.4324/9781003466192-11

Severity	Scope		
	Isolated	Pattern	Widespread
Immediate jeopardy to resident health or safety	J	K	L
Actual Harm that is not immediate jeopardy	G	H	I
No actual harm with the potential for more than minimal harm that is not immediate jeopardy	D	E	F
No actual harm with a potential for minimal harm	A	B	C

Figure 7.1 Scope and Severity of Nursing Home Deficiencies.[2]

Source: Centers for Medicare & Medicaid Services. This figure depicts a rectangle diagram that illustrates nursing home survey deficiency types including scope and severity; labeled from A to L and whether isolated, a pattern, or widespread and ranging from no actual harm to immediate jeopardy utilized by the Centers for Medicare & Medicaid Services in the United States.

The CMS provides the regulatory guidelines for LTC facilities in the United States and is part of the Department of HHS. The Code of Federal Regulations 1987a and 1987b are regulations facilities must comply with to maintain compliance and remain certified. And, 1987c are regulations that the state must follow when conducting investigations or survey processes.

A 2022 article in HHS public access titled, "Reforming Nursing Home Financing, Payment, and Oversight" by Rachel M. Werner MD, PhD, et al., that discusses both LTC and post-acute care in the industry focuses on three areas: LTC financing, nursing home payment, and transparency and accountability in funding and payment, further explaining that any comprehensive nursing home reform must include the establishment of a federal LTC benefit that would expand access and advance equity for all people who need LTC, whether or not it is nursing home care.[3] And, that care for long-stay residents in nursing homes should be paid under alternative payment models that use global capitation or other payment mechanisms that hold nursing homes accountable, versus the per diem payment systems currently in place.[4] In addition, the payment initiatives for post-acute care in nursing homes could be extended to all conditions, in order to hold hospitals financially accountable for post-acute spending and patient-centered outcomes.[5]

Of the 15,000 facilities in the United States, Medicare and Medicaid-certified skilled and LTC homes—92% are certified by both programs[6]. The vast majority of nursing homes are for-profit (70%), non-profit facilities encompass 24% of all nursing homes, and government-owned facilities are at 6%.[7]

Infections in elder care homes account for approximately half of all transfers to hospitals and are a significant source of morbidity and mortality among the elderly population. Nursing homes in the United States are mandated to have an IPC program to prevent the spread of infections and outbreaks and to provide a safe, sanitary, and comfortable environment for clients. At a minimum, an infection control program in US LTC institutions must contain the following elements:

1. Policies, procedures, and practices that promote consistent adherence to evidence-based infection control practices.
2. Program oversight including planning, organizing, implementing, operating, monitoring, and maintaining elements of the program and ensuring that the interdisciplinary team is involved in IPC.
3. Have an IP, as the coordinator of the infection control program.
4. Perform surveillance, process and outcome, monitoring, data analysis, documentation, and reporting of infections as required by state and federal regulations.
5. Provide education, including IPC practices.
6. Perform antibiotic reviews to determine the appropriateness of medications prescribed.

The CDC provides guidance to HHS for infection mitigation during pandemics.

COVID-19-Related Regulatory Improvement Strategies

On October 21, 2022, the Biden-Harris Administration announced new steps to improve the quality of care in nursing homes, due to the COVID-19 pandemic. One of the strategies implemented was a more aggressive enforcement for worst-performing nursing homes. The Special Focus Facilities (SFF) Program announced that they would increase penalties for nursing homes in the program that fail to improve, utilizing escalating penalties for violations. And, nursing homes even after graduating from the SFF program would be closely monitored for compliance for three years to maintain quality of care. It was also announced that there would be an increase in technical assistance for facilities in the SFF program, like support through CMS Quality Improvement Organizations.[8]

In March 2023, the Governmental Accountability Office (GAO) released recommendations based on a study conducted related to US nursing homes and the COVID-19 pandemic titled, *COVID-19 in Nursing Homes: Experts Identified Actions Aimed at Improving Infection Prevention and Control*. The actions that GAO felt that the Department of HHS should enhance in nursing homes, included developing staffing solutions, strengthening mandatory

IPC training, increasing IPC assistance to facilities, strengthening the use of non-monetary enforcement actions, ensuring that there is consistency in the guidance provided, incentivizing IPC research, and strengthening emergency preparedness.[9]

In 2020, CMS released the Long-term Services and Supports (LTSS) rebalancing toolkit Fact Sheet to support states in their efforts to expand and enhance home and community-based services to assist in achieving a more equitable balance in LTC spending and services delivered relative to institutional care. The toolkit identifies promising state models and practices for strengthening state infrastructure to increase transitions from institutional settings to community-based settings, prevent or delay institutionalization, and improve community living for individuals eligible for Medicaid.[10]

Canada-Federal and Provincial Governments

There are approximately 2,076 nursing homes in Canada, which are both publicly (46%) and privately owned (54%) and are governed by provincial/territorial legislation; jurisdiction over health and healthcare is a shared responsibility.[11] Funding for the healthcare provided in LTC in Canada consists of 73% of the costs being covered under provincial, territorial, and municipal plans, and 23% of the costs are covered by resident out-of-pocket payments or private insurance plans. LTC in Canada is considered an extended healthcare service.

Annual inspections (resident quality inspections) of nursing homes are varied in Canada, as each province sets its own standards and regulations. A 2021, annual survey conducted by the HSO, revealed that ensuring the provision of high-quality care in elder care facilities was a top priority of concern. The survey revealed that 67.3% of respondents did not feel that LTC homes in Canada were providing safe, reliable, and high-quality care.[12]

In Canada, the Public Health Agency of Canada provides guidance to the provincial and territorial public health efforts in monitoring, preventing, and controlling healthcare-associated infections. Each province develops their own infection control regulations; there is no one unified IPC regulatory system in Canada for the LTC industry.

Ontario

The Ministry of Health conducted annual nursing home inspections in Ontario until 2016, when a model was implemented that transitioned inspections to a Resident Quality Inspection Intensive (RQI) and RQI lite, the RQI Intensive was to be performed in every elder care home at least every three years through the Long-Term Care Home Quality Inspection Program. It has been perceived by some individuals that when any inspection was conducted in a nursing home (complaint, infection control, etc.), it could qualify as an annual inspection process, and therefore inspections have not been conducted proficiently.

New Brunswick

The government of New Brunswick believes that protecting the health, safety, and well-being of LTC residents is a priority. Regulatory requirements are provided in the Standards Manual and the Nursing Home Act for nursing homes. The Department of Social Development conducts annual inspections through Regional Liaison Officers, and they typically take two days to complete. Nursing homes in New Brunswick are also inspected by the Department of Public Safety, the Office of the Fire Marshall.[13]

Quebec

The MSSS performs inspections in residential elder care homes in Quebec that are currently being conducted every four years, and LTC facilities are inspected every three years. A private seniors' residence is a rental facility that is occupied or designed to be occupied mainly by people aged 65 years or over and where various services are offered, such as nursing care, meal services, housekeeping services, and recreational services.

The designation "private seniors' residence" is reserved for residences that hold a certificate of compliance issued by the Government of Québec, which means that the facility complies with rules to ensure the health and safety of its residents. Current regulations related to elder care are identified in the "Act Respecting Health and Social Services and Long-Term Care." Figure 7.2 illustrates the number of nursing homes in specific Canadian Provinces.

Nova Scotia

In Nova Scotia, the Department of Health and Wellness provides licensing for nursing homes under regulations in the "Homes for Special Care Act Regulations and the Long-Term Care Program Requirements." Elder care facilities are required to have two inspections annually in the Nova Scotia Province. Yet in April 2022, there were 39 LTC facilities handling COVID-19 outbreaks according to Barbara Adams, Minister of Seniors and Long-Term Care.[15]

COVID-19-Related Regulatory Improvement Strategies

The HSO and the Canadian Standards Association (CSA) Group were tasked with coming up with standards to improve the quality of care in LTC homes across Canada. The HSO focused on the care itself and the CSA on the physical

Number of Long-Term Care Homes in Canadian Provinces

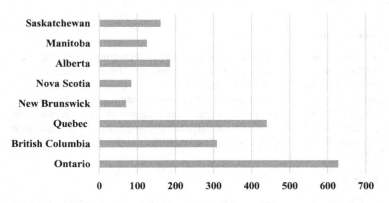

Figure 7.2 Canadian Number of LTC Facilities by Province.[14]

Source: Canadian Institute for Health Information. This illustrates a bar graph with a vertical axis listing provinces in Canada and a horizontal axis of numbers from 0 to 700, showing the number of nursing homes with Ontario having over 600 facilities and New Brunswick under 100.

infrastructure. While the new standards are voluntary, health experts say that they will not do the job unless LTC homes adopt all of them without exceptions.[16]

"This is very much a kind of all-or-nothing thing. This is basically what the standard of care needs to be," said Dr. Samir Sinha, director of geriatrics at Sinai Health and the University Health Network in Toronto and chair of the HSO technical committee that drafted the standards. "My greatest fear is that if we don't take these standards to heart and make sure that they are the basis of inspections, enforcements, quality improvements and accountability . . . I'm worried that these standards will just sit on the shelf."[17]

The two sets of standards are meant to complement each other. They go beyond pandemic preparedness and address everything from preventing falls and maintaining flexible meal schedules (some LTC residents went without meals during staff shortages over the course of the pandemic), to end-of-life care and emergency plans for catastrophic events.[18]

Ontario

In 2021, due to COVID-19, it was announced that 193 new inspection staff would be hired and there would be a new and improved proactive annual inspection of nursing homes launched. The government has a plan to fix LTC that is built on three pillars: improving staffing and care; protecting residents through better accountability, enforcement, and transparency; and building modern, safe, comfortable homes for seniors.[19] The Fixing Long-Term Care Act of 2021 sets standards through the *Resident's Bill of Rights* that states, "Every resident has the right to live in a safe and clean environment."

The Long-Term Care Homes Act of 2007 in Ontario provided IPC guidelines for this province that were carried over to the 2021 newly implemented Long-Term Care Homes Act. The IPC program must include daily monitoring to detect the presence of infection in residents of the LTC home and measures to prevent the transmission of infections.[20] Infection Prevention and Control Canada (IPC) incorporated in 1976 provides education, communication, networking, and advocacy for its LTC home members.

Quebec

In 2021, it was identified that more staff were needed to increase annual inspections of residential elder care facilities with a plan implemented to improve the quality of care for residents by improving governmental monitoring. The MSSS posted 19 new positions for inspectors in résidences pour aînés (RPAs), or private seniors' residences, as there were only seven inspectors to serve over 1,000 homes in the province.[21] As well, the evaluation of increased inspections for LTC facilities is being conducted.

United Kingdom—CQC

In the United Kingdom, there were a total of 17,598 elder care providers—residential care homes (12,471 total) and nursing homes (5,127 total) in August 2021.[22] It is suggested that England provides the majority of these care environments with residential operators consisting of around 10,000 establishments and nursing homes with around 5,000 facilities. Self-funders comprise approximately half of care home residents in this region, the remainder are state-funded, and costs for care are paid by the local authority.

The CQC established in 2009 is a branch of the Department of Health and Social Care in the United Kingdom. They inspect residential care homes and nursing homes in England. Fundamental standards for elder care consist of person-centered care, dignity and respect, consent, safety, safeguarding from abuse, food and drink, premises and equipment, complaints, good governance, staffing, fit and proper staff, duty of candor, and the display of ratings. The organization conducts both comprehensive inspections and focused inspections to implore quality of care for care home recipients.

All LTC facilities in this geographic area are inspected at least once every three years. The CQC website identified ratings for 15,028 providers in October 2022. In 2021, the percentage of ratings revealed that overall it was perceived adequate healthcare was being provided in England as demonstrated in Figure 7.3.

The Department of Health provides education and best practice resources for IPC in elder care homes. A Health and Social Care Act: Code of Practice sets out what registered providers of health and adult social care services need to follow to sustain compliance with the CQC standards for cleanliness and IPC. Compliance criteria include the following:

1. Systems to monitor and manage the prevention and control of infections.
2. Provide and maintain a clean and appropriate environment.
3. Provide accurate information on infections.
4. Ensure early identification of infections and prompt proper treatment.
5. All employees need to provide care that deters and prevents the spread of infections.
6. Provide adequate isolation facilities.
7. Maintain adequate access to lab support.
8. Follow policies and procedures that prevent the spread of infections.
9. Ensure that education is provided to care workers on the prevention and control of infections.

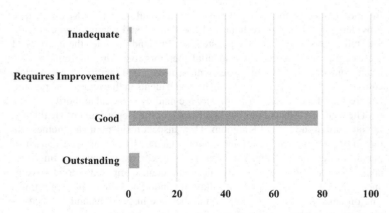

2021 UK Care Homes: Percentage of Perceived Quality of Care

Figure 7.3 Perceived Quality of Care in Care Homes in the United Kingdom[23]

Source: Statista. This bar graph has a horizontal axis of percentages 0–100% and a vertical axis listing perceptions of nursing homes in Canada from inadequate to outstanding, with the majority of responses being above 75% for good.

The educational materials provided also cover monitoring and reporting of infections, risk assessment, surveillance, outbreak recognition, root cause analysis, visitors, occupational health, chain of infection, and standard infection control protocols.

Scotland

Care Inspectorate (Social Care and Social Work Improvement Scotland) evaluates the quality of care in nursing homes in Scotland. Regulations are provided by the Public Services Reform (Scotland) Act 2010 and the National Care Standards, and compliance is evaluated with annual inspections. A comparison study in Scotland between the years 2011 and 2021 revealed that the number of elder care homes decreased by 20%, the resident census decreased by 11%, and the number of registered facilities declined by 5%.[24]

Ireland

Northern Ireland has the Regulation and Quality Improvement Authority (RQIA) that was established under the Health and Personal Social Services (Quality Improvement and Regulation) Order 2003. Each provider of elder care services is inspected two times per year to ensure quality of life, care, environment, management, and care standards.

COVID-19-Related Regulatory Improvement Strategies

Of 2,934 IPC inspections carried out prior to the end of 2022 in England, almost half were rated as substandard care—the survey results were either inadequate, which consisted of 237 homes, or required improvement that entailed 1,224 homes inspected by the CQC.[25]

A Department of Health and Social Care spokesperson said: "In the Spring we will publish a plan for adult social care system reform, setting out how we will build on this progress over the next 2 years."[26]

Additionally, all new care homes must be inspected by the CQC within 6 to 12 months of opening. If the report shows the care home is providing an inadequate service, another CQC inspection will happen within six months. For a rating of "requires improvement," a further inspection will take place after 12 months, and if rated good or outstanding, it can be as long as five years before the next inspection. Receiving a rating of inadequate means the care home is performing badly and the CQC has taken action against the organization or person who runs it. The Adult Social Care System Reform strategies published in April 2023 aim to relaunch the Adult Social Care Survey and Survey of Adult Carers in England in 2025.[27]

Spain—Ministry of Health

Established in 2007, the first LTC system was developed with the approval of LAW 39/2006-Law of the Promotion of the Autonomy and Care of People in a Dependent Situation, which led to the System for Autonomy and Care for Dependence. The Ministry of Health, Social Services, and Equality (a department of the government of Spain) is responsible for the policy on health and provision/regulation of healthcare in elder care homes.

Spain has both state-run care homes and privately owned nursing homes. The leading care home operators in 2021 were as follows: Domus Vi—20,000 beds, Orpea—9,000 beds, Vitalia—8,000 beds, Ballelsol—7,000 beds, and Sanitas—7,000 beds.[28] LTC providers receive governmental subsidies to make the expense of healthcare more affordable for recipients. Spain does set standards concerning staffing ratios in elder care facilities, and their nursing homes are inspected annually according to some sources, but on the Ministry of Health website, it states that healthcare providers will be periodically evaluated.

The ECDC provides assistance to the Ministry of Health, Social Services, and Equality in Spain. The Ministry of Health has been addressing IPC in healthcare facilities through various programs since 2008. The National IPC Manuals were launched as part of a collaborative effort between the Ministry of Health, the National Coordinating Committee to Combat Antimicrobial Resistance, the PAHO/WHO, and local stakeholders. E-manuals are available for all healthcare providers in Spain—Guidelines for Cleaning, Disinfection, and Sterilization of Medical Devices; Environmental Cleaning for Prevention of Infections in all Health Care Facilities; and IPC—Policies Guidelines for Health Care Services.

Italy—Aziende Sanitaire Locali

The Aziende Sanitaire Locali (regional level) is the Italian Ministry of Health that is responsible for administrative operations related to public healthcare in Italy; this branch works under the National Healthcare Services. In 2021, there was a total of approximately 323,000 beds available in residential and semi-residential facilities (547 beds for every 100,000 inhabitants).[29] The nursing home sector in Italy is highly fragmented, consisting mostly of small operators, with many facilities managed by charities, co-operatives, and church-run organizations. The operator with the highest number of beds in Italy is Segesta (Korian group) with 7,000 beds (estimated figure), followed by KOS (Cir group) with 6,200 beds, and S.O. Holding with around 5,600.[30] Currently, there is no integrated quality assessment system at the national level, but some regions have implemented their own indicators as a monitoring and management tool.

As stated previously, the major focus in Italy for quality assurance is in hospitals. The National Law 52/1985 details IPC for hospitals that could be applicable to nursing/elder care homes. The law directs healthcare facilities to implement strategies for the prevention and surveillance of facility-acquired infections and education of employees. The Ministry of Health, WHO, and the ECDC provided assistance and guidance to healthcare facilities in Italy and were all actively participating in strategies to control the spread of SARS-CoV-2 during the pandemic.

COVID-19-Related Regulatory Improvement Strategies

It has been identified that a national reform through the Ministry of Health that establishes better national standards for regionally managed LTC systems, measuring quality of care by developing inspection processes to assess minimum levels of healthcare and patient safety standards in elder care facilities, and the development of new models of aged care should be implemented to improve elderly quality of life.[31]

In addition, in Italy, there is also no public reporting at the national level on the performance of nursing homes or home care agencies. The major focus for quality assurance, systems improvement, data collection, safety, and education/training encompasses hospitals. The Ministry of Health addressing the implementation of public reporting of LTC facility performance levels could enhance the quality of care in Italian nursing homes also.

France—National Authority for Health

Haute Autorité de Santé (HAS—National Authority for Health) is an independent public body in France set up by the government in 2004 to improve the quality of patient care and equity in healthcare. The 17 Agence Régionale de Santé or ARS (Regional Health Agencies) overseen by the Ministry for Solidarity and Health conduct inspections on health, safety, operations, and medical procedures and practices. As of 2021, Korian and Orpea were the leading nursing home operators in France. During this year, Korian operated 30,000 care home beds and Orpea managed 24,000 beds. The third biggest LTC facility operator in France was Domus Vi, with 20,000 beds in 2021.[32] Nursing homes are regulated under Article L. 311–1 et seq, **code** de l'**action** sociale et des familles (CASF), French Family and Social Action Code.

The country of France has one of the oldest-aged populations in the world. In January 2020, it was estimated that about 1,459,000 people over 60 years of age living at home were deemed to be dependent, and 584,000 people living in institutions could be added, meaning that there are just over two million dependent older people in France. Projections indicate that this number will increase by 200,000–410,000 (+15% to +33%) by 2030. France could have around four million senior citizens with a loss of autonomy in 2050, representing 16.4% of people aged 60 years or over.[33]

A national infection control program was set up in France from 1993 to 2004 to strengthen infection prevention activities at the local, regional, and national levels; improve surveillance; and address antibiotic-resistant microbes. Santé Publique France, Départment des Maladies infectieuses (SpF-DMI) was created in 2016 to address infection surveillance, control, and prevention; health promotion; and research and education. SpF-DMI works with the Regional Health Agencies to address IPC in France. Also, the Ministry for Solidarity and Health follows guidelines and recommendations from the WHO and the ECDC.

COVID-19-Related Regulatory Improvement Strategies

In a policy paper, *Integrated Care for Older People in France in 2020: Findings, Challenges, and Prospects,* the French Society of Geriatrics and Gerontology defined *integration* as a process designed to overcome the fragmentation of services for vulnerable people, requiring an inter-sectoral and multilevel approach, further elaborating on the definition Dennis Kodner and Corinne Kyriacou included that *integration* is a set of techniques and organizational models designed to create connectivity, alignment, and collaboration within and between the treatment and care sectors at the funding, administrative, and/or provider levels. The goals were to enhance quality of care and quality of life, patient satisfaction, and system efficiency for patients with complex problems cutting across multiple sectors and providers.[34]

Germany—Federal Ministry of Health

Social and private LTC insurance became mandatory in 1995 to cover LTC costs. The LTC strengthening acts of 2015–2017 assisted in establishing a more deinstitutionalization (outpatient before inpatient) mindset for this country. In Germany, the majority of elder care is provided in private or residential care homes versus institutional nursing homes. Citizens have a choice to receive cash for informal care or obtain professional care in the home, or clients can obtain a combination of both services.

The German Federal Ministry of Health oversees the insurance programs, quality of healthcare systems, and the protection against infection act. Along with multiple other responsibilities since its establishment in 1961, the branch addresses LTC services and needs. The 2001, LTC Quality Assurance Law assists with establishing standards of care in German nursing homes. A care home supervisory authority (competent care home regulatory body) is responsible for supervising and advising care homes, including nursing homes, with a main focus on protecting the interests and needs of the occupants, and can perform on-site inspections as part of the monitoring process. In addition, the Medical Review Board of the Statutory Health Insurance Funds can conduct inspections, monitor regulations, and provide oversight of all elder care homes. Germany's plan to reform nursing homes will be elaborated on in more detail in the next chapter.

A 2001 Protection Against Infection Act (with ongoing amendments) was established to prevent communicable diseases, detect infections at an early point and time, and prevent the spread of infections. The Robert Koch Institute is the federal branch responsible for disease control and prevention in Germany that is connected with the ECDC. Germany's Ministry of Health and Medical Advisory Board assist with IPC compliance in LTC facilities.

Most countries have implemented some type of changes with regard to regulatory statutes in nursing homes due to the COVID-19 pandemic, as discussed in this chapter. However, the provision of regulatory guidelines and the entities that enforce these standards in elder care homes varies greatly from country to country. Some countries have no one organization responsible for quality of healthcare in LTC facilities at a national level yet rely on each state or province to set their own set of standards. This leaves avenues for disruption of healthcare services provision, due to no clear uniform standard of guidelines established in their facilities. In emergency situations, such as a pandemic, this could potentially exacerbate consequences for elder care recipients.

Notes

1 US Department of Health and Human Services: Data Brief. (2019). Trends in deficiencies at nursing homes show that improvements are needed to ensure the health and safety of residents. Office of Inspector General. A-09–16–02021. p. 1.
2 Centers for Medicare & Medicaid Services. (2022). SFF scoring methodology. www.cms.gov/Medicare/Provider – Enrollment-and-Certification/ CertificationandComplianc/Downloads/SFFSCORINGMETHODOLOGY.pdf. (accessed October 25, 2023).
3 Werner, Rachel, MD, PhD, et al. (2022). Reforming nursing home financing, payment, and oversight. *New England Journal of Medicine.* 386(20). https://doi.org/10.1056/NEJMp2203429. https://pubmed.ncbi.nlm.nih.gov/35551508. (accessed December 26, 2023). pp. 1869–1871.
4 Werner, Rachel, MD, PhD, et al. (2022). Reforming nursing home financing, payment, and oversight. *New England Journal of Medicine.* 386(20). https://doi.org/10.1056/NEJMp2203429. https://pubmed.ncbi.nlm.nih.gov/35551508/. (accessed December 26, 2023). pp. 1869–1871.
5 Werner, Rachel, MD, PhD, et al. (2022). Reforming nursing home financing, payment, and oversight. *New England Journal of Medicine.* 386(20). https://doi.org/10.1056/NEJMp2203429. https://pubmed.ncbi.nlm.nih.gov/35551508/. (accessed December 26, 2023). pp. 1869–1871.
6 Boccuti, Cristina. (2015). *Reading the Stars: Nursing Home Quality Ratings, Nationally and by State.* Kaiser Family Foundation. www.kff.org/report-section/reading-the-stars-nursing-home-quality-star-ratings-nationally-and-by-state-issue-brief/. (accessed July 16, 2022). pp. 3, 6.

7 Boccuti, Cristina. (2015). *Reading the Stars: Nursing Home Quality Ratings, Nationally and by State.* Kaiser Family Foundation. www.kff.org/report-section/reading-the-stars-nursing-home-quality-star-ratings-nationally-and-by-state-issue-brief/. (accessed July 16, 2022). pp. 3, 6.

8 The White House. (2022). Fact sheet: Biden-Harris administration announces new steps to improve quality of nursing homes. www.whitehouse.gov/briefing-room/statements-releases/2022/10/21/fact-sheet-biden-harris-administration-announces-new-steps-to-improve-quality-of-nursing-homes/. (accessed October 10, 2023).

9 Government Accountability Office. (2023). COVID-19 in nursing homes: Experts identified actions aimed at improving infection prevention and control. www.gao.gov/assets/gao-23-105613.pdf. (accessed October 10, 2023).

10 CMS. (2020). Long-term services and supports (LTSS) rebalancing toolkit fact sheet. https://www.cms.gov/newsroom/fact-sheets/long-term-services-and-supports-ltss-rebalancing-toolkit-fact-sheet. (accessed December 26, 2023).

11 Canadian Institute for Health Information. (2021). Long-term care homes in Canada: How many and who owns them? www.cihi.ca/long-term-care-homes-in-canada-how-many-and-who-owns-them#. (accessed July 21, 2022).

12 Health Standards Organization. (2021). Health Standards Organization (HSO) is pleased to release the What We Heard Report #1: Findings from HSO's Inaugural National Survey on Long-Term Care. www.healthstandards.org/general-updates/health-standards-Organization-pleased-release-heard-report-1-findings-hs. (accessed July 21, 2022).

13 Department of Social Development. (2022). Inspection of nursing homes, Government of New Brunswick. https://www2.gnb.ca/content/gnb/en/departments/social_development/nursinghomes/content/inspection-of-nursing-homes. (accessed July 21, 2022).

14 Canadian Institute for Health Information. (2021). Long-term care homes in Canada: How many and who owns them? www.cihi.ca/long-term-care-homes-in-canada-how-many and-who-owns-them#. (accessed July 21, 2022).

15 Patil, Anjuli. (2022). 39 long-term care facilities in N.S. dealing with COVOD-19 outbreaks. *CBC News.* https://www/cbc.ca/news/canada/nova-scotia/39-n-s-long-term-care-facilities-dealing-with-covid-19-1.6418827. (accessed July 22, 2022).

16 Roman, Karina. (2023). New voluntary standards released for long-term care homes devastated by the pandemic. *CBC News.* www.cbc.ca/news/politics/long-term-care-canada-standards-pandemic-1.6730780. (accessed October 10, 2023).

17 Roman, Karina. (2023). New voluntary standards released for long-term care homes devastated by the pandemic. *CBC News.* www.cbc.ca/news/politics/long-term-care-canada-standards-pandemic-1.6730780. (accessed October 10, 2023).

18 Roman, Karina. (2023). New voluntary standards released for long-term care homes devastated by the pandemic. *CBC News.* www.cbc.ca/news/

politics/long-term-care-canada-standards-pandemic-1.6730780. (accessed October 10, 2023).
19 Ministry of Health News. (2021). Ontario launching new and improved inspections program for long-term care. https://news.ontario.ca/en.release/1001041/ontario-launching-new-and-improved-inspections-program-for-long-term-care. (accessed July 21, 2022).
20 Ontario Legislative History. (2007). Long-term care homes act, Chapter 8. www.ontario.ca/laws/statute/07l08?search=Long-Term+Care+Homes+Act,+2007. (accessed November 5, 2023).
21 CBC News. (2021). Quebec aims to increase inspections in private seniors' residences with dozens more inspectors. www.cbc.ca/news/canada/montreal/quebec-quadruples-number-of-inspectors-in-retirement-homes-1.6265359. (accessed October 10, 2023).
22 Michas, Frederic. (2021). Number of residential care homes and nursing homes in the United Kingdom in 2021. *Statista*. www.statista.com/statistics/1236800/residential-care-homes-and-nursing-homes-in-the-united-kingdom/. (accessed October 8, 2022).
23 Michas, Frederic. (2021). Quality level of care dispensed in care homes in the UK 2021. *Statista*. www.statista.com/statistics/quality-level-of-care-in-care-homes-in-the-uk-2021. (accessed October 8, 2022).
24 Public Health Scotland. (2021). Care home census for adults in Scotland. www.publichealthscotland.scot/care-home-census-for-adults-in-scotland. (accessed October 8, 2022).
25 Corker, Sarah. (2023). Almost half of care homes inspected in England found to be failing, figures show. www.itv.com/news/2023-01-24/almost-half-of-all-care-homes-inspected-in-england-found-to-be-failing. (accessed October 10, 2023).
26 Corker, Sarah. (2023). Almost half of care homes inspected in England found to be failing, figures show. www.itv.com/news/2023-01-24/almost-half-of-all-care-homes-inspected-in-england-found-to-be-failing. (accessed October 10, 2023).
27 Department of Health and Social Care. (2023). Policy paper: Next steps to put people at the heart of care. https://www.gov.uk/government/publications/adult-social-care-system-reform-next-steps-to-put-people-at-the-heart-of-care/next-steps-to-put-people-at-the-heart-of-care. (accessed October 10, 2023).
28 Michas, Frederich. (2022). Leading care home operators in Spain in 2021, by number of beds. *Statista*. https://statista.com/statistics/1236814/care-home-operators-with-most-beds-in-spain/. (accessed October 9, 2022).
29 Media Relations. (2023). The leading private healthcare operators in Italy: Profitability declining, but revenues back above pre-covid levels. www.areastudimediobanca.com/sites/default/files/2023-04/Press_Release_Healthcare_2023_2.pdf. (accessed November 5, 2023).
30 Media Relations. (2023). The leading private healthcare operators in Italy: Profitability declining, but revenues back above pre-covid levels. www.areastudimediobanca.com/sites/default/files/2023-04/Press_Release_Healthcare_2023_2.pdf. (accessed November 5, 2023).

31 Cepparulo, Alessandra, and Giuriato, Luisa. (2022). The residential healthcare for the elderly in Italy: Some considerations for post COVID-19 policies. *European Journal of Health Economics.* 23(4). www.ncbi. nlm.nih.gov/pmc/articles/PMC8549427. (accessed October 11, 2023). pp. 671–685.
32 Michas, Frederich. (2022). Leading care home operators in France in 2021, by number of beds. *Statista.* https://statista.com/statistics/1236804/leading-care-home-operators-in-france-2021-by-number-bed/. (accessed October 11, 2022).
33 Bajeux, Emma, et al. (2021). Integrated care for older people in France in 2020: Findings, challenges, and prospects. *International Journal of Integrated Care.* 21(4). https://doi.org/10.5334/ijic.5643. (accessed October 11, 2023). pp. 1–12, 16.
34 Bajeux, Emma, et al. (2021). Integrated Care for Older People in France in 2020: Findings, Challenges, and Prospects. *International Journal of Integrated Care.* 21(4). https://doi.org/10.5334/ijic.5643. (accessed October 11, 2023). pp. 1–12, 16.

8 Government Strategies for Healthcare Delivery Improvement Processes in Long-Term Care

In September 2021, the US Government, Biden-Harris Administration released *American Pandemic Preparedness: Transforming Our Capabilities*, stating that the United States must fundamentally transform its ability to prevent, detect, and rapidly respond to pandemics and high-consequence biological threats, describing goals for the country under five pillars:

- Transforming our Medical Defenses, including dramatically improving vaccines, therapeutics, and diagnostics.
- Ensuring Situational Awareness about infectious-disease threats, for both early warning and real-time monitoring.
- Strengthening Public Health Systems, both in the United States and internationally to be able to respond to emergencies, with a particular focus on protecting the most vulnerable communities.
- Building Core Capabilities, including PPE, stockpiles and supply chains, biosafety and biosecurity, and regulatory improvement.
- Managing the Mission, with the seriousness of purpose, commitment, and accountability of an Apollo Program.[1]

President Biden hosted a virtual *Global COVID Summit: Ending the Pandemic and Building Back Better* on September 24, 2021, which included participation by representatives from more than 100 governments and more than 100 leaders from international organizations, the private sector, civil society, academia, and other stakeholders. The main focus at this meeting was the COVID-19 vaccination process that was addressed by United Nations Secretary, General Antonio Guterres; WHO Director, General Dr. Tedros Adhanom-Ghebreyesus; Republic of South Africa's President, Matamela Cyril Ramaphosa; European Commission President, Ursula von der Leyen; Republic of Indonesia President, Joko Wildodo; World Trade Organization Director, General Dr. Ngozi Okonjo-Iweala; Canada's Prime Minister, Justin Trudeau; and Gavi, the Vaccine Alliance Chief executive Officer, Dr. Seth Berkly.[2]

DOI: 10.4324/9781003466192-12

Beyond vaccines, as part of strengthening the health systems in the United States, efforts to improve staffing in nursing homes are ongoing and central to advancing the quality of elder care.

Staffing

New steps to improve the quality of care in nursing homes were announced by the Biden-Harris administration in October 2022. The plan addressed more resources to support good-paying union jobs in nursing home care. The Department of HHS and the Department of Labor highlighted new funds available to obtain this goal, including:

- $80 million in grant funding for a variety of workforce stakeholders
- $13 million in grants to expand nursing education and training
- Additional federal funds to support the nursing workforce pipeline including YouthBuild, the National Dislocated Worker Grant Program, and WORC Initiative Grants[3]

WORC is the Workforce Opportunities for Rural Communities program within the Department of Labor. The Biden-Harris Administration also called for establishing minimum staffing requirements in nursing homes.

The US Department of HHS through the CMS in September 2023 proposed a new rule for minimum staffing requirements in nursing homes, calling for nursing home residents to have a minimum of three hours of direct care each day, including 30 minutes of care from an RN and 2.5 hours from a nurse's aide (CNA). Also the CMS proposal would require all nursing homes to have a RN on site 24 hours per day/seven days per week. US HHS Secretary, Xavier Beccera said,

> Establishing minimum staffing standards for nursing homes will improve resident safety and promote high quality care so residents and their families have peace of mind.[4]

This proposed rule builds on the President's historic Action Plan for Nursing Home Reform launched in the 2022 State of the Union address.

Additionally, CMS announced a national campaign to support staffing in nursing homes. As part of the HHS Workforce Initiative, CMS will work with the Health Resources and Services Administration and other partners to make it easier for individuals to enter careers in nursing homes, investing over $75 million in financial incentives, such as scholarships and tuition reimbursement. This staffing campaign builds on other actions by HHS and the Department of Labor to build the nursing workforce.[5]

Kaiser Family Foundation

The Kaiser Family Foundation released a brief with regard to the new CMS staffing requirements, identifying key takeaways as follows:

- Among all nursing facilities, fewer than one in five could currently meet the required hours for RNs and nurse aides, which means over 80% of facilities would need to hire nursing staff.
- 90% of for-profit facilities would need to hire additional nursing staff compared with 60% of non-profit and government facilities.
- The percentage of nursing facilities that would meet the requirements in the proposed rule varies from all in Alaska (100%) to nearly none in Louisiana (1%).[6]

The implementation of the new rule will be instituted in phases, with phase one taking effect 60 days after publication of the rule that entails facility-wide staffing assessments and evaluation of the needs of each resident to establish required staffing levels. The second phase that requires an RN on duty 24 hours/day, 7 days/week will take effect two years after publication of the rule for urban facilities and three years for rural nursing facilities. And, the third phase is the number of nursing (HPRD) hours per resident day (0.55 RN and 2.45 CNA) increasing the HPRD to 3.48.[7] It is perceived that increasing staffing ratios will improve quality of care and establish a stronger foundation in nursing homes, preparing for future public health emergencies.

Another part of the plan for regulatory improvement is increasing accountability and transparency in nursing homes, and this is regarded as crucial.

Transparency and Accountability

On February 12, 2023, the Biden-Harris Administration proposed a rule that would increase transparency of nursing home ownership. The rule would require nursing homes to disclose to CMS and states additional ownership and management information, including private equity and real estate investment trust definitions. CMS Administrator, Chiquita Brooks-LaSure, stated, "If finalized, this rule would strengthen our ability to examine ownership types, including private equity and real estate investment trusts."[8]

It is suggested that the rule will assist in an increased understanding of the nursing home market.

And, Director Rohit Chopra at the Elder Justice Coordinating Council meeting in 2021, stated,

Private equity investors typically seek to purchase assets, often using significant amounts of debt financing, to ramp up operating profits before selling. And, private equity investments regarding LTC in the US have increased more than 1,900% over the past two decades: from less than $5 billion in 2000 to $100 billion in 2018, raising the question of whether for-profit incentives are misaligned with serving our seniors well.[9]

CMS also proposes to require states to collect and report on compensation for workers as a percentage of Medicaid payments for those working in nursing homes and intermediate care facilities.[10] These policies build on CMS' proposals to support compensation for direct care workers in home- and community-based settings and to publish Medicaid data on average hourly pay rates for home care workers. This enhanced transparency will aid efforts to support and stabilize the LTC workforce across settings.[11] Workforce adversities in LTC were also addressed by the National Academy of Sciences through a recently conducted comprehensive study.

National Academy of Sciences

Additionally, in 2022, a 604-page report (it is the first study of the nursing home industry in 35 years) by the National Academy of Sciences, Engineering, and Medicine concludes, "the way in which the United States finances, delivers, and regulates care in nursing home settings is ineffective, inefficient, fragmented, and unsustainable."[12] *The National Imperative To Improve Nursing Home Quality: Honoring Our Commitment to Residents, Families, and Staff* identifies seven broad goals and recommendations that provide a framework to improve the quality of care in US nursing homes including workforce, transparency, financing, and survey/enforcement.

Other Governmental Identified Reform Strategies

Other nursing home reform initiatives in the October 2022, Biden-Harris Administration plan are cracking down on illegal debt collection, incentivizing quality performance through Medicare and Medicaid funding, improving families' ability to comparison shop, and ensuring pandemic preparedness.[13] In 2021, the LTC service supports in the United States totaled $467.4 billion.[14]

Additional announcements from CMS and the HHS Office of the Inspector General (HHS-OIG) made in September 2023 are systems that would increase transparency; enhance enforcement of existing standards; increase accountability; and ensure safe, high-quality, and dignified care for people living in nursing homes. The proposed reforms are to increase audits of nursing homes' staffing; improve nursing home inspections; ensure taxpayer dollars go toward safe, high-quality care; crack down on inappropriate antipsychotic prescribing practices and risks; and enhance resident safety during emergencies.[15]

Australian Government

The Department of Health and Aged Care in Australia has implemented several aged care reforms since the COVID-19 pandemic that aim to put older Australians first, improving quality, safety, and choice in aged care.

1. Under the trusted, safe, and high-quality care section in the recommendations, there is a wage increase for both in-home and community aged care providers, more stay-at-home care packages, extension in the disability support for older individuals, and implementation of a one single assessment process.[16]
2. New processes to ensure equitable access include the increase in funding for the National Aboriginal and Torres Strait Islander Flexible Aged Care Program, improving access to culturally safe care for First Nations elders, assigning an interim First Nations Aged Care Commissioner, and introducing a First Nations assessment workforce.[17]
3. The government aims to place older people at the center by delivering a new Aged Care Act that embeds choice in residential aged care, institutes new incentives for general practitioners to improve primary care, and implements policies reflecting that no person under the age of 65 years will reside in residential aged care.[18]
4. In addition, there are government processes to promote sustainable care for an aging population through the Fair Work Commission that will fund 11.3 billion AUD over four years to maintain staffing stability. An improved Aged Care Taskforce will be implemented and more funding will be provided for residential aged care services. There will be an expansion of viability support programs for providers and provisions of 12.9 million AUD to the Aged Care Prudential Reform Program through the Aged Care Quality and Safety Commission. In addition, the government plans to reduce the aged care provision ratio from 78 to 60.1 places per 1,000 people (70 years and older) over three years.[19]
5. The Australian government will also institute processes that measure success in the sector by building a strong regulatory framework for aged care, boosting monitoring and compliance, and expanding and aligning aged care worker screening.[20]

Additional national aged care reforms to improve accountability and transparency in the aged care sector established through the Aged Care and Other Legislation Amendment (Royal Commission Response) Act 2022 in Australia include the aged care 24/7 RN requirement that was implemented on July 1, 2023, a code of conduct for aged care, new consent arrangements around restrictive practices, strengthened aged care quality of standards, and provision of reformed care standards webinars.[21]

Reformed In-Home Aged Care

In addition, the Australian government will initiate reforming in-home aged care through the new Support at Home Program that will begin on July 1, 2025. Current and future engagements for the in-home care program include the following:

- From July to December 2023, the Aged Care Taskforce conducted independent engagements, giving expert advice on a range of design details, including the service list.
- In September 2023, consulting was initiated on how respite care will be delivered under the new program.
- From September to November 2023, there was engagement with the First Nations communities on developing a culturally safe, trauma-informed pathway to in-home aged care.
- Between September and November 2023, there was a consultation on assistive technology and home modification to develop an inclusion list and advise on the needs of people with progressive conditions.
- In October 2023, there was conduction of a study on the provision of higher levels of in-home aged care to support people to remain independent in their own homes longer.
- On December 14, 2023, there was the fifth reforming in-home aged care webinar to update on the Support at Home program and the single assessment system for aged care.
- From December 2023 to early 2024, the Independent Health and Aged Care Pricing Authority conducted a pricing study to determine fair and efficient prices for in-home aged care.[22]

The Australian government, like many other countries, is assessing avenues that would allow for the elderly to stay at home for longer periods, establishing more effective IPC strategies by reducing the risk of cohabitation environments.

UK Government

All four countries in the United Kingdom have instituted reform programs for adult social care. *The People at the Heart of Care* white paper published in December 2021 put forth a ten-year plan for improvement in adult social care in England that encompassed €2.1 billion in funding to establish system reforms. The vision puts people at the heart and has three objectives:

- People have choice, control, and support to live independent lives.
- People can access outstanding quality and tailored care and support.
- People find adult social care fair and accessible.[23]

Included in the plan are activities that improve access to care and support, recognize skills for careers in care, improve digital transformation in adult social care, improve transparency and accountability, support people to be independent at home, drive innovation and improvement, and join up people to support people and carers. In the plan from October 2023 onward, there will be a cap of €86,000 that any individual will have to spend on their personal care over a lifetime.

Wales

In Wales, the white paper *Rebalancing Care and Support* published in January 2021 addresses healthcare partners, balancing the market for care provision and improving commissioning practices. The rebalancing of the national framework will set the terms through which services for people who are in need of care and support are commissioned by developing a set of common commissioning practices and a range of fee methodologies that commissioners will be required by law to use, simplifying procurement and ensuring greater visibility of service standards through the following:[24]

- A national framework for commissioned care and support (Code of Practice)
- A national office for care and support
- Strengthening of regional partnership board arrangements
- Introducing new legislation to achieve the vision set out in the Social Services and Well-being Act 2014
- Developing a national framework for commissioning social care that will rebalance care and support[25]

Scotland

Scotland is in the process of developing the legal basis for a National Care Service through the legislature; the bill was introduced to the Scottish Parliament in June 2022. The purpose is to have social care shifted from local government to Scottish ministers by 2026. And, Care Boards will be developed at the local level to shape social care. The Scottish Government states,

> we want everyone to have access to consistently high-quality social care support across Scotland, whenever they might need it. Our goal is to

future-proof the social care sector for generations to come-and for people coming into the profession.[26]

Ireland

The Department of Health launched the *Reform of Adult Social Care in Northern Ireland* in January 2022. A consultation on adult social care addressed 48 proposed actions to obtain a reform in the adult social care system over the next ten years. Some of the areas addressed are funding and charging, integrated care, market regulation, workforce, training, safe staffing, legislation, domiciliary care, and care homes.[27]

Canadian Government

The HSO in Canada released new national standards to improve LTC facilities. The Standards Council of Canada, HSO, and the CSA Group worked collaboratively to develop two new national standards for LTC. Under the new proposed guidelines that build on the previous standards from 2020, the criteria for resident-centered care, safe practices, and a healthy and competent workforce have been added. The new standard provides LTC home residents, teams, and the workforce, leaders, and governing bodies with guidance on:

- Providing evidence-informed, resident-centered care that values compassion, respect, dignity, trust, and a meaningful quality of life
- Working in a team-based way to deliver high-quality care that is culturally safe and trauma-informed to meet residents' goals, needs, and preferences
- Enabling a healthy and competent LTC home workforce and healthy and safe working conditions
- Upholding strong governance practices and a culture that is outcome-focused and committed to continuous learning and quality improvement[28]

The content of the standard is structured into the following sections: governing LTC home's strategies, activities, and outcomes; upholding resident-centered care; enabling a meaningful quality of life for residents; ensuring high-quality and safe care; enabling a healthy and competent workforce; and promoting quality improvement. The standard also integrates the principles of equity, diversity, and inclusion. In addition to the above, the standard also provides:

External assessment bodies with evidence-informed content and a quality/safety blueprint that can be used in assessment programs and by decision makers to guide policy development and requirements to ensure the delivery of high-quality, resident-centered care, and enable a healthy and competent workforce.[29]

Nursing Retention Forum

The Government of Canada hosted a Nursing Retention Forum on June 14, 2023, led by Canada's Chief Nursing Officer, Dr. Leigh Chapman-bringing together the nursing community, employers, and frontline workers from across the country to discuss the current health workforce crisis including strategies to address and improve nursing retention. The Government of Canada will continue to work with provinces, territories, the Coalition for Action for Health Workers, and other key stakeholders to identify solutions to long-standing health workforce challenges so that nurses and other health workers across Canada can continue their critical work of keeping Canadians healthy and safe.[30]

Nurses are the backbone of our healthcare system, yet too many in Canada are struggling with their mental health, feeling burned-out, overworked, distressed, and unappreciated, causing them to leave their jobs entirely. Co-developing a retention toolkit will allow the nursing community to contribute first-hand to making changes in our health care system, including improving mental health supports to help nurses stay mentally, emotionally, and spiritually healthy, so that they can keep supporting us.

The Honourable Carolyn Bennett Canada's Minister of Mental Health and Addictions and Associate Minister of Health[31]

Italian Government

In Italy, both the Ministry of Health and the Ministry of Labour Market and Social Affairs have been working on plans to achieve goals to reform LTC since the summer of 2021. In particular, the latter Ministry created an ad hoc "LTC Reform Commission," chaired by L. Turco, a former Social Affairs and Healthcare Minister. And, the "Turco Commission" produced a Reform Proposal, which was formally presented to Prime Minister M. Draghi in January 2022; some of the recommendations are as follows:

1. Introduction of basic social levels of LTC provision (Livelli essenziali delle prestazioni sociali), which are based on the right to access a set of services
2. Greater integration between social and healthcare services in relation to LTC
3. Strengthening of the coordination among municipalities for joint planning and joint commissioning of LTC (the so-called "Ambiti Territoriali Sociali")

4. Strengthening of home care services, also improving the use of digitalization and e-health
5. Introduction of several different types of assisted living solutions for frail elderly people (co-housing, etc.), which have been tried out over recent decades in many Italian municipalities, but have not received national specific codification and formal recognition
6. Strengthening of both respite care services and support for caregivers[32]

As of October 2023, no additional documentation as to how the process has progressed in relation to the implementation of reforms is available, but again, there is a strong recommendation for the improvement of in-home care services in Italy.

German Government

The German Federal Health Minister, Jens Spahn, presented a nursing reform bill that was passed by the Bundestag (German Parliament) on June 11, 2021. The most important points of the bill are mandatory collectively agreed salaries for nursing staff and a gradual reduction of the co-payment for residents in nursing homes.[33]

From September 1, 2022, only nursing homes that pay nursing and social support staff according to collective agreements will be allowed to operate. The resulting higher costs are to be offset by an annual federal subsidy of € one billion, as well as a 0.1% increase in contributions for childless persons to the LTC insurance system. The goals of the reform are to provide better working conditions, financial relief in nursing homes, and better quality of care.

"In order for nursing homes to hire more nursing staff, we will prescribe a nationwide staffing ratio that will allow for further hiring of additional nursing staff," the Federal Ministry of Health informed.[34]

Gross Domestic Product

It is estimated that approximately 1.5% of the gross domestic product (GDP) is allocated for LTC in OECD countries.[35] The GDP is the total value of goods produced and services provided in a country during one year. Figure 8.1 depicts percentages of GDP in specific countries.

Countries providing more funding to nursing homes during the pandemic likely increased the GDP percentages from 2020 to 2023. Globally, the average government expenditure on LTC is less than 1% of the GDP. Most African countries spend 0% of their GDP on LTC, with the exception of South Africa, which spends 0.2% of its GDP.[37] In the Americas, expenditure ranges from 1.2% of the GDP in the United States to 0.6% in Canada and 0% in Latin

2019 Percentage of GDP Allocated for LTC

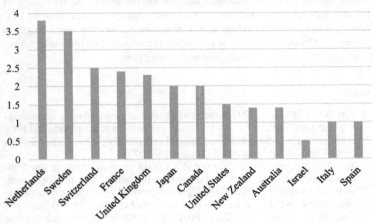

Figure 8.1 GDP for LTC 2019.[36]

Source: OECD. This is a column graph that has a vertical axis illustrating percentages 0–4% and a horizontal axis listing specific countries, showing the percentage of GDP allotted for LTC with Israel being the lowest at 0.5% and the Netherlands being the highest at above 3.5%.

American countries.[38] In Asia and the Pacific, New Zealand spends the most on LTC (1.3%) and Australia spends the least (0%), while countries such as China, India, and Indonesia spend less than 1% of GDP on LTC.[39]

In Europe, public spending on LTC is expected to rise from 1.7% of the GDP in 2019 to 2.5% of the GDP in 2050 on average across the EU, with large variations between member countries.[40] In a scenario assuming some upward convergence among Member States, EU-27 expenditure could more than double to 3.4% of the GDP in 2050. Assuming that social protection coverage remains at current levels, it is projected that, in the EU, an absolute increase in the number of recipients (of all ages) of public LTC services and benefits will be as follows: (a) home care recipients from 6.9 million in 2019 to 8.2 million in 2030 and 10.5 million in 2050 and (b) residential care recipients from 4.5 million to 5.1 million in 2050.[41]

The aging population in all countries is one of the reasons why reform of elder care services needs to be viewed more seriously. In most countries, the elderly would prefer to stay at home and avoid institutionalization, if possible. This should be one of the core reasons to evaluate and expand on different strategies to improve possibilities for in-home gerontological care services throughout the world. Many countries have already initiated evaluating and implementing strategies to assist in deinstitutionalization of nursing homes, recognizing that the morbidity and mortality related to the COVID-19 pandemic require reforms to be implemented that support the health and well-being of this vulnerable population globally. The coming years will reveal how the LTC industry adapts, how the elderly and their representatives perceive changes in this sector of healthcare, and how governments continue to institute and enforce reforms to improve elder health care and nursing homes.

Notes

1 The White House. (2021). American pandemic preparedness: Transforming our capabilities. www.whitehouse.gov/wp-content/uploads/2021/09/American-Pandemic-Preparedness-Transforming-Our-Capabilities-Final-For-Web.pdf. (accessed October 15, 2023).
2 The White House. (2021). Global COVID summit: Ending the Pandemic and building back better. www.whitehouse. gov/briefing-room/statements-releases/2021/09/24/global-covid-19-summit-ending-the-pandemic-and-building-back-better/. (accessed October 15, 2023).
3 The White House. (2022). Fact sheet: Biden-Harris administration announces new steps to improve quality of nursing homes. www.whitehouse.gov/briefing-room/statements-releases/2022/10/21/fact-sheet-biden-harris-administration-announces-new-steps-to-improve-quality-of-nursing-homes/. (accessed October 15, 2023).
4 US Department of Health and Human Services. (2023). HHS proposes minimum staffing standards to enhance safety and quality in nursing homes. https://www.hhs.gov/about/news/2023/09/01/hhs-proposes-minimum-staffing-standards-enhance-safety-quality-in-nursing-homes.html. (accessed November 5, 2023).
5 US Department of Health and Human Services. (2023). HHS proposes minimum staffing standards to enhance safety and quality in nursing homes. https://www.hhs.gov/about/news/2023/09/01/hhs-proposes-minimum-staffing-standards-enhance-safety-quality-in-nursing-homes.html. (accessed November 5, 2023).
6 Burns, Alice, et al. (2023). What share of nursing facilities might meet proposed new requirements for nursing staff hours? www.kff.org/medicaid/issue-brief/what-share-of-nursing-facilities-might-meet-proposed-new-requirements-for-nursing-staff-hours/. (accessed October 16, 2023).
7 Burns, Alice, et al. (2023). What share of nursing facilities might meet proposed new requirements for nursing staff hours? www.kff.org/medicaid/issue-brief/what-share-of-nursing-facilities-might-meet-proposed-new-requirements-for-nursing-staff-hours/. (accessed October 16, 2023).
8 US Department of Health and Human Services. (2023). Biden-Harris administration continues unprecedented efforts to increase transparency of nursing home ownership. www.hhs.gov/about/news/2023/02/13/biden-harris-administration-continues-unprecedented-efforts-to-increase-transparency.html. (accessed June 18, 2023).

9 Consumer Financial Protection Bureau. (2021). Remarks of Director Rohit Chopra at the elder justice coordination council meeting. www.consumerfinance.gov/about-us/newsroom/remarks-director-rohit-chopra-elder-justice-coordinating-council-meeting/. (June 18, 2023).

10 US Department of Health and Human Services. (2023). HHS proposes minimum staffing standards to enhance safety and quality in nursing homes. www.hhs.gov/about/news/2023/09/01/hhs-proposes-minimum-staffing-standards-enhance-safety-quality-in-nursing-homes.html. (accessed October 15, 2023).

11 US Department of Health and Human Services. (2023). HHS proposes minimum staffing standards to enhance safety and quality in nursing homes. https://www.hhs.gov/about/news/2023/09/01/hhs-proposes-minimum-staffing-standards-enhance-safety-quality-in-nursing-homes.html. (accessed October 15, 2023).

12 The National Academy of Sciences. (2022). The national imperative to improve nursing home quality: Honoring our commitment to residents, families, and staff. https://nap.nationalacademies.org/resource/26526/Nursing_Homes_Highlights.pdf. (accessed November 5, 2023).

13 The White House. (2022). Fact sheet: Biden-Harris administration announces new steps to improve quality of nursing homes. https://www.whitehouse.gov/briefing-room/statements-releases/2022/10/21/fact-sheet-biden-harris-administration-announces-new-steps-to-improve-quality-of-nursing-homes/. (accessed October 15, 2023).

14 Congressional Research Services. (2023). Who pays for long-term care services and supports? https://crsreports.congress.gov,/product/pdf/IF/IF10343. (accessed October 15, 2023). p. 1.

15 US Department of Health and Human Services. (2023). HHS proposes minimum staffing standards to enhance safety and quality in nursing homes. www.hhs.gov/about/news/2023/09/01/hhs-proposes-minimum-staffing-standards-enhance-safety-quality-in-nursing-homes.html. (accessed October 15, 2023).

16 Department of Health and Aged Care. (2023). Aged care reforms. www.health.gov.au/our-work/aged-care-reforms. (accessed June 19, 2023).

17 Department of Health and Aged Care. (2023). Aged care reforms. www.health.gov.au/our-work/aged-care-reforms. (accessed June 19, 2023).

18 Department of Health and Aged Care. (2023). Aged care reforms. www.health.gov.au/our-work/aged-care-reforms. (accessed June 19, 2023).

19 Department of Health and Aged Care. (2023). Aged care reforms. www.health.gov.au/our-work/aged-care-reforms. (accessed June 19, 2023).

20 Department of Health and Aged Care. (2023). Aged care reforms. www.health.gov.au/our-work/aged-care-reforms. (accessed June 19, 2023).

21 Aged Care Quality and Safety Commission. (2023). National aged care reform. www.agedcarequality.gov.au/reforms. (accessed June 19, 2023).

22 Department of Health and Aged Care. (2023). Engagements for reforming in-home aged care. www.health.gov.au/our-work/reforming-in-home-aged-care/engagements-for-reforming-in-home-aged-care. (accessed October 16, 2023).

23 Department of Health and Social Care. (2023). Next steps to put people at the heart of care. www.gov.uk/government/publications/adult-social-care-system-reform-next-steps-to-put-people-at-the-heart-of-care/next-steps-to-put-people-at-the-heart – of-care. (accessed June 19, 2023).

24 Welsh Government. (2021). Rebalancing care and support. www.gov.wales/sites/default/files/consultations/2021-01/consutation-document.pdf. (accessed June 19, 2023).

25 Welsh Government. (2023). Rebalancing care and support: Consultation document. www.gov.wales/sites default//files/consultations/2023–05/consultation-document.pdf. (accessed June 19, 2023).

26 Scottish Government. (2023). Social care. www.gov.scot/policies/social-care-national-care-service/. (accessed June 19, 2023).

27 Department of Health. (2022). Reform of adult social care Northern Ireland: Consultation document. www.health-ni.gov.uk/consultation-reform-adult-social-care. (accessed June 19, 2023).

28 Health Standards Organization. (2023). About the standard and how it was developed. https://longtermcarestandards.ca/about-standard. (accessed June 20, 2023).

29 Health Standards Organization. (2023). About HSO's standards. https://health-standards.org /standard/long-term-care-services-can-hso21001–2023-e/. (accessed June 20, 2023).

30 Health Canada. (2023). Government of Canada and Chief Nursing Officer hosted the Nursing Retention Forum to address health workforce challenges. www.canada.ca/en/health-canada/news/2023/06/government-of-canada-and-chief-nursing–officer-hosted-the-nursing-retention-forum-to-address-health-workforce-challenges.html. (accessed June 20, 2023).

31 Health Canada. (2023). Government of Canada and Chief Nursing Officer hosted the Nursing Retention Forum to address health workforce challenges. www.canada.ca/en/health-canada/news/2023/06/government-of-canada-and-chief-nursing–officer-hosted-the-nursing-retention-forum-to-address-health-workforce-challenges.html. (accessed June 20, 2023).

32 Pavolini, Emmanuele. (2022). *On the Verge of a Long-term Care Reform in Italy?* ESPN Flash Report 2022/41. European Social Policy Network (ESPN). Brussels: European Commission. pp. 1, 2.

33 Forum. (2021). Nursing care reform in Germany to provide better working conditions and financial relief in nursing homes. www.stiegelmeyer-forum.com/en/articles-reports/nursing-care-reform-in-germany-to-provide-better-working-conditions-and-financial-relief-in-nursing-homes.html. (accessed October 16, 2023).

34 Forum. (2021). Nursing care reform in Germany to provide better working conditions and financial relief in nursing homes. www.stiegelmeyer-forum.com/en/articles-reports/nursing-care-reform-in-germany-to-provide-better-working-conditions-and-financial-relief-in-nursing-homes.html. (accessed October 16, 2023).

35 OECD. (2021). Long-term care spending and unit costs. www.oecd-ilibrary.org/sites/cb584fa2-en/index.html?itemId=/content/component/cb584fa2-en. (accessed June 24, 2023).

36 OECD. (2021). Long-term care spending and unit costs. www. oecd-ilibrary.org/sites/cb584fa2-en/index.html?itemId=/content/component/cb584fa2-en. (accessed June 24, 2023).
37 Costa-Font, Joan and Raut, Nilesh. (2022). *Global Report on Long-Term Care Financing.* Report for World Health Organization. https://extranet. who.int/kobe_centre/sites/default/files/WHO_Report_Draft_Juen2022_r. pdf. (accessed October 16, 2023).
38 Costa-Font, Joan, and Raut, Nilesh. (2022). *Global Report on Long-Term Care Financing.* Report for World Health Organization. https://extranet. who.int/kobe_centre/sites/default/files/WHO_Report_Draft_Juen2022_r. pdf. (accessed October 16, 2023).
39 Costa-Font, Joan and Raut, Nilesh. (2022). *Global Report on Long-Term Care Financing.* Report for World Health Organization. https://extranet. who.int/kobe_centre/sites/default/files/WHO_Report_Draft_Juen2022_r. pdf. (accessed October 16, 2023).
40 Costa-Font, Joan, and Raut, Nilesh. (2022). *Global Report on Long-Term Care Financing.* Report for World Health Organization. https://extranet. who.int/kobe_centre/sites/default/files/WHO_Report_Draft_Juen2022_r. pdf. (accessed October 16, 2023).
41 Costa-Font, Joan, and Raut, Nilesh. (2022). *Global Report on Long-Term Care Financing.* Report for World Health Organization. https://extranet. who.int/kobe_centre/sites/default/files/WHO_Report_Draft_Juen2022_r. pdf. (accessed October 16, 2023).

Index

Printed in the United States
by Baker & Taylor Publisher Services

Printed in the United States
by Baker & Taylor Publisher Services